RECIPES FOR HEALTH

Low Blood Sugar

RECIPES FOR HEALTH

Low Blood Sugar

Over 100 recipes for overcoming hypoglycaemia

MARTIN BUDD & MAGGIE BUDD

Thorsons
An Imprint of HarperCollins*Publishers*

Thorsons
An Imprint of HarperCollins*Publishers*
77–85 Fulham Palace Road,
Hammersmith, London W6 8JB
1160 Battery Street,
San Francisco, California 94111–1213

Published by Thorsons 1995
1 3 5 7 9 10 8 6 4 2

A catalogue record for this book
is available from the British Library

ISBN 0 7225 2913 9

Printed in Great Britain by
HarperCollins Manufacturing, Glasgow

Contents

Foreword

I AM VERY pleased to have the opportunity of introducing this book which I know will be a source of help to a great many people. I have had the privilege of working in close collaboration with Martin Budd at the Basingstoke Clinic over the past twenty years and we have shared in the often demanding task of treating and supporting perhaps a thousand victims of what Mr Budd appropriately called the '20th century epidemic'. His experience in the field of Functional hypoglycaemia makes this latest book, written jointly with Maggie Budd, clinically authoritative. The many recipes, which have been formulated to provide the increased protein/carbohydrate ratio fundamental to successful treatment, will give real practical help.

We have never been fully aware just why hypoglycaemia became such a neglected clinical backwater. Be that as it may, the publication of Mr Budd's first book in 1981 brought a steady flow of letters from patients throughout the UK complaining of a wide range of symptoms which the author had described as 'low blood sugar syndrome'. Regrettably, the majority of these patients had been unable to obtain the help they sought. Although seminars were organised by The Basingstoke Clinic, there are still not enough practitioners experienced in the diagnosis and treatment of functional hypoglycaemia.

This book will therefore fill a need, both in providing self-help to patients in suitable cases, and in drawing attention to a neglected area of clinical practice.

Keith Lamont
Basingstoke, Hants

Note: In December 1984 The Basingstoke Clinic came under new management and the original team became dispersed.

Introduction

M OST OF US have experienced symptoms of hypoglycaemia or low blood sugar. These may include weakness, tremors, dizziness, palpitations, anxiety and hunger. The commonest triggers for these unpleasant symptoms are stress or sudden shock, unaccustomed exercise, a missed or delayed meal, excessive coffee or alcohol intake, and in women, the 4–5 day premenstrual effect. Frequently there exists a combination of 2 or more of these factors.

Although a sudden fall in the blood sugar can be responsible for some of the above symptoms, the more unpleasant acute symptoms associated with low blood sugar are in fact caused partly by the release into the blood of the hormone adrenalin. This hormone, which is released by the paired adrenal glands situated over each kidney, serves to convert into glucose the carbohydrate reserves held in the liver, and known as glycogen. In this way undesirably low levels of glucose in the blood are quickly corrected. Although this adrenal compensation is triggered when the blood glucose is too low, the same response can occur when the blood glucose level falls too quickly.

Adrenalin is also released to help the body combat stress. In addition to the blood sugar surge, this hormone increases the heart rate and raises the blood pressure. The rate of respiration is also increased; in fact the whole metabolism is 'revved-up'. This has been termed the 'flight or fight' response, and can be compared to pulling out the choke on a car, causing an increase in available fuel and accelerating the engine.

The hunger experienced with low blood sugar is usually expressed as a sugar craving (particularly pre-menstrually), and all the symptoms rapidly improve after taking sugar in food or drink. If the various components of the sugar-regulation system are working efficiently our body chemistry is rapidly normalised. This phenom-enon is known as transient hypoglycaemia, and such infrequent and temporary slumps in the blood sugar level do not normally require special diets or treatment.

FUNCTIONAL HYPOGLYCAEMIA

Unfortunately there are those who suffer a more chronic, severe and reoccuring form of low blood sugar, known as functional hypoglycaemia. This condition was first described in the late 1920s by an American doctor named Seale Harris. His contemporaries Banting and Best had recently discovered and refined the hormone insulin for the treatment of diabetes. Insulin-dependent diabetics can occasionally overdose on insulin, causing a sudden undesirable fall in the blood sugar. This was termed a 'hypo effect', and caused symptoms including faintness, dizziness, anxiety and if severe, a temporary collapse and unconsciousness.

Dr Harris observed that several of his non-diabetic patients were experiencing very similar symptoms to patients attending the new diabetic clinics. This led him to conclude that if non-diabetics were suffering 'hypos' (or insulin shock), then perhaps there existed a medical condition that was opposite in character to high blood sugar in diabetes. He called this new condition hyperinsulinism, (excess insulin in the blood), and assumed that just as diabetics suffer an insulin deficiency resulting in high blood sugar, there are those who suffer an excess causing low blood sugar. Although high and low blood sugar appear to be opposite conditions, they are both caused by defective or inefficient blood sugar regulation.

Dr Harris stated that an overworked pancreas could be the cause of hyperinsulinism and this condition could in many cases precede diabetes. Overactivity of the body's systems and organs with subsequent exhaustion and inefficiency is a common pattern in disease. As this type of low blood sugar is caused by faulty function and not by damage or disease, it is now known as functional hypoglycaemia. The term hyperinsulinism has been reserved to describe the more serious organic problems that cause excessive insulin production.

ORGANIC HYPOGLYCAEMIA

Apart from functional hypoglycaemia and hypoglycaemia of diabetes, there are other types of hypoglycaemia, termed Organic. These are caused by a variety of diseases including pancreatic tumours, liver disease and other fairly obscure glandular disorders. This more serious side of low blood sugar highlights the need for accurate diagnosis and effective treatment. Surgery may be essential for the relief of these non-functional types of hypoglycaemia.

HOW SUGAR IS METABOLISED

Together with starches and fibre, sugar is one of the three main carbohydrates in food. It is the body's chief fuel and an important source of energy.

Chemically speaking, carbohydrates are made up of units called monosaccharides. These units can exist by themselves, in pairs (disaccharides), or in long chains (polysaccharides). Monosaccharides and disaccharides are called simple sugars, while polysaccharides, which include starches and cellulose (fibre), are called complex carbohydrates. The commonest simple sugars are glucose (blood sugar, and also found in fruit and honey), fructose (fruit sugar), galactose (found in milk), sucrose (table sugar), lactose (found in milk), and maltose (found in malted barley).

All sugars and starches are broken down during digestion to form the monosaccharide glucose, used for energy. Any spare sugar is converted into glycogen, a polysaccharide stored in the liver and muscle tissues. Glycogen in the liver is stored ready for conversion back to glucose as needed. However the muscle glycogen cannot be sent to the blood to be turned into glucose. It is only available as a fuel for the muscle tissue. When the liver and muscle tissues reach saturation, any surplus carbohydrate not required for immediate energy needs is converted into fat and stored in the fatty tissue. When the liver's glycogen stores are depleted, the body uses protein from food or muscle tissue as a secondary source of energy and converts it into glucose.

If we eat unrefined complex carbohydrates such as brown rice, pulses, wholemeal bread and pasta the conversion of these large long chain polysaccharides to glucose in the blood is gradual, and our tissues and blood contain only enough sugar for normal functional requirements.

Unfortunately the Western diet tends to be high in refined carbohydrates and sugar-rich foods such as cakes, biscuits and white bread. The long chain molecules of the natural complex carbohydrates are absorbed slowly, but the small molecules of the refined, processed carbohydrate products are rapidly absorbed through the membranes lining the mouth and stomach. This can result in a sudden excessive surge of glucose into the blood, which triggers the insulin response.

This rapid and usually frequent increase in the blood sugar stresses the sugar-regulation system. This control system includes the pancreas, the liver and the endocrine

Introduction

5

glands (the adrenal glands, the thyroid and pituitary glands). A high-sugar diet can lead to a 'hair trigger' situation, whereby an overstimulated pancreas releases more and more insulin, finally leading to functional hypoglycaemia.

Fructose (fruit sugar), unlike many other sugars, does not require insulin control. For this reason diabetics are allowed it in moderation. When eating whole fruit, our appetite tends to regulate the amount of fructose we can consume. If we eat two or three apples our hunger is rapidly satisfied and we soon feel very full. Although we can consume the sucrose (table sugar) equivalent of 5–10 pounds of apples in a very short time, if we eat chocolate, cakes, ice-cream or sucrose itself, our blood sugar levels may be badly upset because our systems have not yet evolved sufficiently to cope with these large amounts of refined carbohydrates. The outcome is likely to result in a tendency for functional hypoglycaemia, with all of its attendant problems.

When discussing low blood sugar, many people assume that the correct treatment is to simply eat more sugar. Unfortunately taking extra sugar merely stimulates further an already oversensitive and overworked pancreas, causing an insulin excess and a further fall in the blood sugar level. Thus the symptoms are aggravated and worsened, showing that consuming sugar as a treatment for low blood sugar can cause a bio-chemical vicious circle, leading to alternating high and low levels of blood sugar.

CONTROLLING BLOOD SUGAR LEVELS

Starches and simple sugars (fructose, lactose etc) and some protein are all initially broken down by the process of metabolism into glucose (blood sugar) which is used to provide energy and assist oxygen transport. Because glucose passes into the blood before being stored in the liver and muscle, a mechanism to control excessive levels in the blood is essential. This control is achieved by specialised cells in the pancreas (known as the Islets of Langerhans), which release the hormone insulin.

Should the blood sugar levels fall too quickly or too low, the brain triggers the adrenal glands to release adrenalin. This stimulates the liver to release stored glycogen, which is converted back into glucose. In this way the blood sugar is normalised.

If we enjoy good health and our metabolism is stable and efficient, these control systems should work well. But an overworked, over sensitive pancreas may produce excessive insulin, leading to low blood sugar. Eventually an abused and weakened pancreas may not provide sufficient insulin and diabetes could result.

WHAT CAUSES FUNCTIONAL HYPOGLYCAEMIA

The causes of functional hypoglycaemia are many and varied, for as you will have read the sugar regulation processes are complex and interdependent. The overconsumption of sugar in food and drink does not automatically lead to low blood sugar or diabetes. Such factors as inheritance, stress, smoking, alcohol, allergies and general poor health all contribute to problems with 'glucose tolerance'.

The main causes are:

- Pancreatic overstimulation, leading to an insulin excess or hyperinsulinism.
- Adrenal underproduction, leading to an adrenalin deficiency or hypoadrenalism.
- Imbalance in the workings of other endocrine glands, in particular the thyroid and pituitary.
- Excessive consumption of sugar in food and drink.
- Excessive use of tobacco, alcohol and caffeine, all of which stress the adrenal glands.
- Inability to handle prolonged or excessive stress, leading to overwork and weakening of the adrenal system, known in America as 'adrenal exhaustion'.
- Food allergies which can be caused or aggravated by low blood sugar.
- Mineral deficiencies: the trace mineral chromium, also known as 'the glucose tolerance factor', is deficient in the soil of many Western countries resulting in a lack of this mineral in our diet. A deficiency in our diet results in blood sugar control becoming less efficient. The minerals zinc, manganese, magnesium and potassium are also helpful in treating low blood sugar.
- Hereditary factors such as general ill-health can contribute to blood sugar problems.

HOW TO TREAT FUNCTIONAL HYPOGLYCAEMIA

This book should not be seen as a self-treatment manual. Readers are urged to seek the advice of a physician experienced in diagnosing and treating blood sugar problems. If functional hypoglycaemia is suspected, a 6-hour glucose tolerance test, with additional blood and/or hair tests, may be necessary to identify the problem and perhaps to eliminate the possibility of more serious illnesses.

Many sufferers of low blood sugar may be required initially to follow a diet that is at least as disciplined and restrictive as a diet prescribed for an unstable diabetic. This particularly applies in the early stages of treatment when patients can experience quite severe swings in their blood sugar levels.

The recipes and diets in this book are more appropriate for the long-term control and maintenance of normal blood sugar, because the generous use of complex carbohydrates in the recipes may not be appropriate when treating severe or early-stage imbalances in the blood sugar levels. In fact, a strict low-starch regime is usually advocated in the initial two or three months of treatment. This serves as a transition from the high-sugar, refined food diet so often followed by hypoglycaemic patients, to the maintenance programme outlined in this book. The diagnosis and treatment of functional hypoglycaemia is described in detail in Martin Budd's other book, *Low Blood Sugar* (see Further Reading).

WHY THIS BOOK IS NEEDED

Over the last twenty years Martin Budd has treated this problem using nutritional medicine, yet many patients have expressed uncertainty over the type of maintenance regime to follow.

Although there are many excellent books available describing the causes and symptoms of low blood sugar, there are very few books that offer detailed treatment requirements for its long-term control. It is hoped that this book will provide a valuable insight into protein variety and meal planning for this widespread but largely ignored health problem.

KEY POINTS FOR PLANNING A LOW BLOOD SUGAR DIET

There are three major considerations when planning the ideal maintenance diet for blood sugar control:

1. The sugar content of food and drink
2. The absorption rate (glycaemic index) of carbohydrates
3. The timing of meals and between-meal snacks

The Sugar Content of Food

The bulk of sugars are derived from cereal grains, pulses, vegetables and fruits. The only sugar of animal origin that we regularly consume is lactose (milk sugar). Western nations consume in excessive of 50kg of sugar (ie sucrose) per person each year.

The type of sugar eaten determines the speed of absorption. This is particularly relevant to those suffering from diabetes or functional hypoglycaemia as the speed of absorption influences the insulin response and the subsequent level of blood sugar.

The Absorption Rate (glycaemic index) of Carbohydrates

The American naturopath Paavo Airola has written '. . . when we eat sugar in the form of natural carbohydrates, our blood and tissues usually contain *only* the amount of sugar needed for normal functions'. This is a very significant statement, because many of us abuse our metabolism by dumping large amounts of rapidly absorbed sugar into our systems. The ideal diet should be low in protein and fat, and high in natural complex carbohydrates. It is only during the last century that our Western diet has changed to one high in refined sugar and animal protein. Unfortunately our digestive system has not yet sufficiently evolved to efficiently deal with such a rapid transition in eating habits. The modern diet has thrown our sugar-regulating organs, digestive enzyme efficiency and bowel health into confusion and imbalance.

The absorption rate of the carbohydrates varies according to their complexity (see page 159). The simple sugars usually present in refined processed foods are absorbed rapidly via the lining of the mouth and stomach. This causes a rush of glucose into the blood. Natural complex carbohydrates are absorbed slowly via the small intestine walls, allowing a gradual conversion to glucose.

If our metabolism is efficient and healthy, the blood sugar surge created by a high-refined food diet is counteracted in two ways:

- Glucose is withdrawn from the circulation by various body tissues for conversion into energy
- Surplus glucose is converted to the polysaccharide glycogen, and stored in the liver and muscle as a reserve energy source

Unfortunately, repeated excessive sugar consumption can defeat our body's blood sugar regulation back-up systems, leading to an imbalance in the blood sugar level. Excessive overworking of the pancreas, liver and adrenal glands can lead to eventual hypoglycaemia, oxygen deficit and adrenal imbalance, causing a wide range of symptoms.

Although this imbalance can also be triggered by stress (caused by adrenal overload and exhaustion), excessive intake of caffeine, nicotine, alcohol and certain drugs, the modern high-sugar refined food diet is undoubtedly the chief culprit.

It is worth noting that the only sugar available to primative man, apart from that found in fruit, vegetables and some cereals, was the sugar found in wild bee honey. This occasional sugar intake would not have challenged our ancestors' blood sugar regulation system.

The Timing of Meals and Between-meal Snacks

The food that we eat provides us with energy, the main source of which is glucose. If we eat regularly and sensibly our blood sugar level will not surge or fall too quickly. When the diet is high in rapidly absorbed sugary food, and high-starch irregular meals, the result is severe fluctuation in the blood sugar levels.

Meals taken regularly every 3–4 hours and largely consisting of slowly absorbed complex carbohydrates with a protein or fat component, will prevent sudden rises and falls in the blood sugar level. This will ensure a reasonably normal appetite level thus avoiding the cravings for sugar, caffeine and alcohol that are frequently triggered by undesirable falls in the blood sugar level.

The night fast can be a problem as many of us do not eat for twelve or more hours after our evening meal. One solution is to have a late supper or a snack just before retiring. Breakfast should be eaten as early in the morning as is convenient. If for various reasons there is a long delay between waking and eating, a glass of natural fruit juice taken on rising will help by providing a natural boost to the blood sugar.

THE MAINTENANCE DIET

There are many factors that influence the amount of refined carbohydrate and sugar permitted in a low blood sugar diet. These include the dieter's weight, activities, age and not least the severity of their problem. As with diabetes, a little trial and error is required to arrive at an enjoyable varied diet that controls the blood sugar.

Body Weight

Using the recipes in this book as a guide, eat as much as your appetite demands and your weight dictates. This applies to main meals and to those all-important snacks between meals. This book is not obsessively concerned with calorie counting. For weight control you may reduce the size of your servings, but not the frequency of eating. It is quite possible to lose weight on a low blood sugar diet. It is essentially low in sugar and moderately low in fats. Conversely those underweight frequently achieve a normal weight as their blood sugar stabilizes.

Cooking Methods

Casserole cooking, steaming, roasting and microwaving are the best methods. Avoid frying protein foods such as meat, fish and poultry and do not boil vegetables. Boiling causes loss of nutrients, in particular the water-soluble B vitamins and vitamin C. Considerable amounts of minerals are also leached from boiled food.

Raw Foods

Most nutritionists and naturopaths advocate a large percentage of raw food in our diet. Wherever possible fruits and vegetables are best eaten uncooked. There are, however, several very important exceptions to this. Some vegetables contain harmful substances such as oxalic acid, which should not be eaten raw in large amounts. Cooking can reduce the harmful substances to safe levels. This advice applies particularly to the mustard family, which includes broccoli, sprouts, cabbage, cauliflower, horseradish, kale, radish, turnip, swede and watercress; and to the lily family which includes asparagus, chives, garlic, onion, leek and shallot. It also applies to rhubarb, although this is always eaten cooked. Many readers will identify vegetables in this list which can cause them indigestion if taken in excess, particularly when eaten raw.

Certain beans, especially soya beans, contain enzymes that can inhibit the body's ability to absorb protein. Although it is unlikely and dangerous to do so, eating these beans in a raw state can cause indigestion with mineral and protein loss as a consequence. Cooking destroys the enzyme inhibitors and facilitates an efficient digestion. The inhibitors can also be removed if the soya beans are soaked in water for 24 hours, with the water changed every 6 hours.

The minerals found in all grains and most dried peas and beans are bound to a substance called phytin or phytic acid. If these foods are eaten sprouted, the minerals are released and benefit the consumer. When the same foods are eaten raw and dried, they are improperly digested and the minerals are wasted, being excreted with the phytin, to which they remain chemically bound.

Baking and cooking cereals releases the minerals (in particular zinc, iron, manganese and magnesium) from their chemical bond allowing them to be efficiently absorbed and utilised. Adding extra bran to refined grain products should be avoided as bran also contains phytin which prevents absorption.

So, to sum up, eat raw food wherever possible. Some vegetables (mustard and lily family) are best steamed or boiled, discarding the water. Grains should be cooked or eaten in their raw, sprouting state.

Foods to Avoid

It is important to avoid sugar-rich foods such as cakes, pastries, sweets, chocolate and biscuits. Also avoid sweet and sour dishes (with sugar) sauces and gravies (when made with refined flour) and canned fruit in heavy syrup.

Fortunately many manufacturers now offer a range of sugar-free products which are widely available.

Many foods contain hidden sugars, as sugar is used in food processing as a preservative in addition to its role as a sweetener. Many canned and processed meats and vegetables contain sugar.

Not surprisingly, confectionery can contain an excessive amount of sugar, as the examples show.

Food	Amount	Sugar equivalent in teaspoonful
Chocolate fudge	100g/4oz	14
Chewing gum	1 stick	3
Chocolate cake	1 medium slice	14
Sponge cake	1 medium slice	6
Doughnut	Small	4
Average biscuit	1 biscuit	2

Food	Amount	Sugar equivalent in teaspoonful
Baked custard	125ml/4fl oz	4
Ice cream	150g/5oz	6
Apple pie	1 medium slice	12
Chocolate sauce	1 teaspoonful	4
Jam	1 tablespoonful	3
Honey	1 tablespoonful	3
Cocoa (all milk)	225ml/8fl oz	5
Coca Cola	1 bottle	4
Liquorice Allsorts	50g/2oz	11
Milk chocolate bar	50g/2oz	8
Fruit yogurt	50g/2oz	4

Drinks

Avoid sugar-rich or caffeine-rich drinks. This includes most alcohol, coffee, tea, soft drinks, colas and the many other drinks with added sugar. Caffeine-free tea and coffee are available. The occasional glass of dry wine *with* food will not be harmful, in fact many red wines contain natural enzymes that assist digestion.

SHOPPING

The Label Trap

Before your first shopping trip, empty your store cupboard look carefully at the tins and packets, and start to learn the art of label reading in the comfort of your own home. You will quickly learn and be amazed by the different names for sugar and how many products actually contain sugar.

Many manufacturers are making more of an effort to produce sugar-free goods. Most of the major supermarkets and stores have nutrition services (see page 161) and can advise you should you have any problems.

However, for the first few weeks you will have to read *all* labels carefully. BEWARE the words, sucrose, glucose, caramel, molasses, dextrose and 'natural sweetener', which is often sugar! Also be alert for the statement 'free of artificial preservatives' – sugar is a natural preservative and is often added to foods, in large quantities.

The greatest label trap is in the dairy section of the supermarket and concerns yogurt and fromage frais. *Heavy* emphasis is made on low-fat or no fat, but further reading of the label discloses sugar. The other pitfall is the 'diet' yogurt or fromage frais that is sugar-free but has attached to the pot a small container of sugar-laden fruit syrup to stir in.

Ingredients are now required to be listed on the food packet or container. These lists are in order of concentration (ie the first ingredient is the main constituent). Should sugar be listed towards the end of a long list, the actual amount of sugar present will be minimal.

So allow yourself plenty of time to explore the shelves in the supermarkets and health shops. Try different supermarkets and health shops as different stores specialise in different product ranges and 'own brands'. On shopping trips remember to take your reading glasses if you need them – it is amazing how small the printing on labels can be!

Sugar-free Products

Jams, sauces and desserts that are sugar-free can be found in supermarkets and health shops. A few cans of fruit can be kept for emergency use but ensure that they are preserved in natural fruit juice *not* syrup.

When using sugar-free products it is worth remembering that sugar has the dual role of flavour enhancer and preservative. Bread made without sugar may need to be frozen in packs of 4–6 slices and biscuits should be kept in an air-tight container. Once opened, bought sugar-free products should be stored in the fridge.

Artificial Sweeteners

Try to avoid the use of artificial sweeteners as they serve only to encourage the desire for sweetness. The only sugar that we recommend to be used in recipes is Dietade Fruit Sugar, a powdered fructose.

Use purchased drinks (and food) containing artificial sweeteners very sparingly. A quote from the Nutritionist Carlton Fredericks would be relevant here: 'I believe that in hypersensitive individuals, the sweet taste of synthetic sweeteners may touch off the pancreas by a kind of conditioned reflex action. If this sounds preposterous, remember that the gallbladder in sensitive persons has been seen to contract when its owner scented food being fried.'

When sugar is reduced or removed from cooking, the dominant sweet taste that frequently masks many subtle natural flavours is removed. With this in mind it is always advisable to buy fresh food in season to ensure maximum flavour, quality and food value.

We must all be aware of the differences in taste and texture when comparing Christmas tomatoes and strawberries with the fresh-picked equivalent from English summer fields. When fruits and vegetables are purchased out of season they are either artificially produced under glass or flown across the world to reach our supermarkets in a fresh state. These foods are usually costly and low in nutrients in contrast to locally grown produce that are sun-ripened and sold without too much of a delay between picking and eating.

The nutritional value of fresh food reduces in proportion to the length of time between picking and eating. An example showing the nutritional differences in oranges has proved that a freshly picked orange can contain up to ten times more vitamin C than a typical supermarket orange, although appearance, size and colour may be identical.

THE RECIPES

The recipes in this book offer a representative selection of appropriate meals and snacks for treating low blood sugar. We felt it essential to provide recipes for snacks and packed lunches in addition to the main meals. The vegetarian and vegan recipes should be of value as it is not always easy to devise sugar-free snacks and meals using only protein from plants.

It is worth mentioning here that soya beans are the highest form of non-animal protein available, hence its use throughout the recipes. With this in mind some of the recipes include additional soya products to increase the protein content. These are chiefly recipes for biscuits, bread and cakes, that are protein-rich, with soya flour included.

Some of these recipes are original, many have been provided by friends, others are our own versions of classic recipes taken from a selection of authors. The section on recommended reading (see page 163) includes most of these books.

Low Blood Sugar and the Family

It is generally recognised by those involved in growing, retailing and cooking food, as well as the professionals who practice nutritional medicine, that a whole-food, high-fibre, low-sugar diet, without excess fat, constitutes the ideal diet. The recipes recommended in this book for the treatment of low blood sugar fulfil all these requirements and can therefore be safely offered to the whole family.

Key Points in Cooking for a Low Blood Sugar Diet

There are of course many more recipes than those in this

book which are suitable for this type of regime.

The four essential requirements for a low blood sugar recipe are:

- Low sugar content (or preferably sugar-free)
- A protein component with each meal (animal or plant protein)
- Whole-grain cereals instead of refined cereals
- Wherever possible and without compromising the flavour, additional soya flour can be added to bread, biscuits and pastry

Low Blood Sugar and Diabetes

Although, on the face of it, the recipes for low blood sugar are very similar to those for diabetics, there are in fact several essential differences. The insulin-dependant diabetic is required to follow fairly precise guidelines for carbohydrate consumption. The guidelines must balance the insulin dosage to avoid high and low sugar levels in the blood. The low blood sugar sufferer is allowed whole complex carbohydrate, but a protein component is essential to facilitate slow absorption of the food.

The low sugar rule is however common to both diabetes and low blood sugar, and for this reason, diabetic cookery books are also recommended (see page 163). These books contain many recipes that are suitable for the low blood sugar patient. Conversely diabetics can safely use the recipes in this book.

Adapting Your Own Recipes to Enhance Protein Content

Experiment with replacing some of the plain flour in recipes with soya flour. You can also replace butter with soya margarine and cows milk with unsweetened soya milk. This will provide a double benefit namely reduced fat and increased plant protein. Unfortunately, you must not assume that a soya product is sugar free – keep reading the labels!

COOKERY NOTES

boxed{V} boxed{Ve} Recipes suitable for vegetarians are marked with a V, and vegan recipes marked Ve. Many recipes marked vegetarian can be converted into vegan by substituting vegan cheese for other cheese and soya margarine for butter etc.

- Follow either metrical or imperial measures for the recipes in this book as they are not interchangeable.
- All spoon measures are level
- Size 2 free-range eggs should be used unless otherwise stated
- Milk is semi-skimmed unless otherwise stated
- Plain flour is used unless otherwise stated
- Herbs are fresh unless otherwise stated

1

Breakfast

For anyone suffering the symptoms of low blood sugar, breakfast is the most important meal of the day. A wholemeal cereal with perhaps the addition of fresh fruit makes an excellent start to the day. For those who do manual work or who are obliged to have a late lunch, an extra protein dish can be added or soya milk can be used in place of cows' milk. Many of the recipes in the chapters on Lunch Snacks and Between-meal Snacks can be easily adapted for breakfast.

There are sugar-free jams and marmalades available for use with wholemeal toast or rolls, with either butter or soya margarine.

HIGH PROTEIN CEREAL

Makes 8–10 servings

Metric/Imperial		American
100g/4oz	soya flour	1½ cups
175g/6oz	rolled oats	¾ cup
2 tbsp	bran	2 tbsp
3 tbsp	wheatgerm	3 tbsp
125ml/4fl oz	vegetable oil	½ cup
25g/1oz	sesame seeds, toasted	¼ cup
25g/1oz	sunflower seeds, toasted	¼ cup
100g/4oz	raisins	⅔ cup

1. Preheat oven to 170°C/325°F/gas mark 3.
2. Mix all the ingredients (except the sesame seeds, sunflower seeds and raisins).
3. Spread the mixture on a non-stick baking tray. Roast for 35–45 minutes, stirring occasionally.
4. Allow the mixture to cool, then add the remaining ingredients.
5. Store in an airtight container.

SIMPLE BASIC MUESLI

Makes 10–12 servings

Metric/Imperial		American
50g/2oz	barley flakes	1¼ cups
50g/2oz	rye flakes	1¼ cups
100g/4oz	oat flakes	1 cup
50g/2oz	wheat flakes	1¼ cups
50g/2oz	raisins	⅓ cup
100g/4oz	rolled oats	1 cup
50g/2oz	mixed nuts, coarsely chopped	½ cup
50g/2oz	sunflower seeds	⅓ cup
1	large eating apple	1

1. Mix all the ingredients in a large bowl.
2. Grate apple into each serving just before eating.

Note

Any fresh fruit can be added to replace the apple, or chopped dried fruit. The oats can be soaked overnight in water for ease of digestion.

TOASTED MUESLI

Makes 25–30 servings

Metric/Imperial		American
700g/1½ lb	rolled oats	1½ lb
225g/8oz	coconut flakes	½ lb
100g/4oz	flaked almonds	1 cup
75g/3oz	sesame seeds	⅔ cup
225g/8oz	barley flakes	½ lb
100g/4oz	roasted buckwheat	8 tbsp
225g/8oz	wheatgerm	½ lb
100g/4oz	sunflower seeds	¾ cup
225g/8oz	mixed dried fruit	½ lb
225g/8oz	sultanas	½ lb
100g/4oz	pumpkin seeds	¾ cup

1. Spread the oats on a non-stick baking tray. Cook in a preheated oven at 180°C/350°F/gas mark 4 for 15 minutes until brown. Stir frequently.
2. Cook the coconut, almonds and sesame seeds in a dry frying pan until golden brown, tossing to avoid burning.
3. Combine all the ingredients and leave to cool. Store in an airtight container.
4. Serve with chopped fresh fruit or natural yogurt.

TRADITIONAL OATMEAL PORRIDGE

Serves 2

Metric/Imperial		American
600 ml/1 pt	water	2½ cups
65g/2½oz	medium oatmeal	⅔ cup
1 tsp	salt	1 tsp

1. Bring the water to a rapid boil in a medium-size saucepan.
2. Sprinkle in the oatmeal gradually, whisking all the time.
3. Bring back to the boil, still whisking.
4. Reduce the heat, cover and cook very gently for 10 minutes.
5. Add the salt and whisk well again, cover and cook for a further 15 minutes.
6. Pour into warm serving bowls; and top with low fat natural unsweetened yogurt and a dried fruit compote.

GRANOLA

Serves 6–8

Metric/Imperial		*American*
450g/1 lb	oat flakes	1 lb
3 tbsp	sunflower oil	3 tbsp
50g/2oz	sesame seeds	1/3 cup
50g/2oz	desiccated coconut	2/3 cup
50g/2oz	chopped hazelnuts	1/2 cup
few drops of	vanilla essence	few drops of
100g/4oz	raisins	2/3 cup

1. Preheat oven to 190°C/375°F/gas mark 5.
2. Mix all the ingredients, except the raisins, in a large bowl.
3. Spread the mixture on a baking tray and cook for 20–25 minutes. Turn the mixture regularly to ensure even roasting.
4. When golden brown, remove from the oven and allow to cool.
5. When completely cold stir in the raisins.
6. Store in an airtight container.

BEANS AND CHEESE ON TOAST

Serves 1–2

Metric/Imperial		American
1–2 slices	wholemeal bread	1–2 slices
200g/7oz	sugar-free baked beans	1 cup
75g/3oz	mature Cheddar cheese, grated	¾ cup
	freshly ground black pepper	

1. Toast the bread on one side only. Set aside.
2. Meanwhile, heat the beans thoroughly, then mix in the cheese.
3. Season with pepper, spread over the untoasted side of the bread and grill until bubbling.

TOASTED SARDINE AND CHEESE SANDWICHES

Makes 4 rounds

Metric/Imperial		American
4	canned sardine fillets	4
50g/2oz	cream cheese or Quark	¼ cup
	salt and freshly ground black pepper	
8 slices	wholemeal or granary bread	8 slices
8–10	crisp lettuce leaves	8–10

1. Drain the sardines, chop well and place in a mixing bowl.
2. Add the cheese and seasoning and stir until thoroughly combined.
3. Spread the mixture over all 8 slices of bread.
4. Place the lettuce over 4 slices then place the remaining 4 slices on top, sardine-side down.
5. Toast on both sides under a preheated hot grill.

SMOKED FISH SCRAMBLE
ON TOAST

Serves 2

Metric/Imperial		American
1 tsp	olive oil	1 tsp
50g/2oz	smoked fish (haddock or kipper), cooked and flaked	1/3 cup
2	eggs, beaten	2
4 tbsp	semi-skimmed milk freshly ground black pepper	4 tbsp
1 tbsp	soft cheese	1 tbsp
2 slices	wholemeal bread	2 slices

1. Heat the oil in a saucepan, add the fish and gently heat for 2–3 minutes.
2. Combine the eggs and milk, season with a little pepper, then add to the pan, stirring continuously.
3. When the mixture has thickened and the eggs are cooked, stir in the cheese and remove the pan from the heat.
4. Toast the bread on both sides. Spread equal quantities of the fish mixture over each piece of toast and serve immediately.

SARDINES ON TOAST

Serves 2–3

Metric/Imperial		American
4	canned sardine fillets in olive oil, drained	4
100g/4oz	butter	½ cup
	lemon juice	
	salt and freshly ground black pepper	
2–3 slices	wholemeal bread	2–3 slices

1. Place the sardines and butter in a small mixing bowl and mash together until thoroughly mixed.
2. Add a squeeze of lemon juice, and season with salt and pepper.
3. Toast the bread on one side. Spread the sardine mixture on the untoasted side, and grill for 4–5 minutes until brown.

WELSH RAREBIT

Serves 2

Metric/Imperial		*American*
4 slices	wholemeal bread	4 slices
100g/4oz	mature Cheddar or Red Leicester cheese, grated	1 cup
1 tsp	mustard powder	1 tsp
1 tsp	Worcestershire sauce	1 tsp
pinch	paprika	pinch

1. Toast the bread on one side only.
2. Place the remaining ingredients in a mixing bowl and mix well together. Spread the mixture over the untoasted sides of the bread.
3. Grill for 3–4 minutes until the cheese browns.

SCRAMBLED EGG AND BACON
TOASTED SANDWICH

Serves 4

Metric/Imperial		American
4 large rashers	lean back bacon, rinded	4 slices
8 slices	wholemeal bread	8 slices
	butter	
2 large	eggs, beaten	2 large
	salt and freshly ground	
	black pepper	
2 tbsp	soured cream	2 tbsp
	Worcestershire sauce	
1 tsp	whole-grain mustard	1 tsp

1. Grill the bacon until crisp, then chop finely.
2. Toast the bread on one side only. Spread butter on the untoasted side.
3. Gently scramble the eggs in a saucepan until creamy.
4. Stir in the bacon and season with salt and pepper. Spread the mixture over the untoasted sides of 4 slices of the bread.
5. Mix together the cream, Worcestershire sauce and mustard, and spread over the remaining 4 slices. Close the sandwiches with the toasted surfaces outwards.

BAKED BEAN SPREAD

Serves 4

Metric/Imperial		*American*
200g/7oz can	no sugar baked beans	1 cup
	freshly ground black pepper	
75g/3oz	low-fat Cheddar cheese, grated	¾ cup

1. Put the baked beans in a mixing bowl, mash well and season with pepper.
2. Add the cheese and mix thoroughly.
3. Use as a sandwich filling, or toast bread on one side and spread on the mixture, then grill until brown and bubbling.

Lunch, Snacks and Sandwiches

For those having lunch at home, these recipes are easy to prepare. And several of the recipes in the chapter on Breakfast would also make suitable lunches. Many of the vegetarian recipes can easily be converted to vegan by replacing the dairy foods with plant foods such as cereals, vegetables, pulses, nuts and seeds.

Packed lunches for school and office can include sandwiches, salads, hot soups, protein drinks, high-protein biscuits, and crudites with dips. Fresh fruit makes an ideal dessert at a lunch time meal.

HIGH PROTEIN PANCAKES

Makes 8–10

Metric/Imperial		*American*
1	egg	1
2 tbsp	soya oil	2 tbsp
125ml/4fl oz	milk	½ cup
50g/2oz	soya flour, sifted	½ cup
50g/2oz	oat flour, sifted	½ cup
1½ tsp	baking powder	1½ tsp
1 tsp	salt	1 tsp

1. Put the egg, oil and milk in a mixing bowl and beat together.
2. Add the flours, baking powder and salt. Stir and blend well.
3. Cook the pancakes, one at a time, on a hot griddle or in a non-stick frying pan until browned on both sides.
4. Serve with butter or sugar-free jam, or sprinkle on grated cheese prior to folding.

COURGETTE AND RED ONION FRITTATA

Serves 4

Metric/Imperial		American
2 tbsp	olive oil	2 tbsp
1	large red onion, thinly sliced	1
3	courgettes/zucchini, cut into matchsticks	3
	salt and freshly ground black pepper	
5	eggs (size 3), beaten	5
75g/3oz	feta cheese, cubed	1 cup
2 tbsp	chopped fresh basil	2 tbsp

1. Heat half the oil in a medium frying pan and cook the onion until soft and lightly browned.
2. Add the courgettes and plenty of seasoning, and continue cooking until golden.
3. Combine the eggs, cheese and basil and season well.
4. Remove the onion and courgette mixture from the pan with a slotted spoon and add to the egg mixture, mixing well.
5. Wipe the pan clean and heat the remaining oil. Add the egg mixture and cook over a low heat, stirring occasionally, until set but not brown.
6. Place the pan under a preheated hot grill to cook the top of the frittata.
7. Serve warm or cold, cut into wedges.

ANCHOVY AND PARMESAN EGGS

Serves 2

Metric/Imperial		American
8	anchovy fillets, drained	8
4	eggs, beaten	4
	freshly ground black pepper	
50g/2oz	butter	¼ cup
2 tbsp	freshly grated Parmesan cheese	2 tbsp

1. Chop the anchovies. Season the eggs with a little pepper.
2. Melt half the butter in a saucepan, reduce the heat and pour in the eggs.
3. With the eggs still slightly liquid, stir in the remaining butter with the cheese and anchovies.
4. Serve on hot buttered toast.

TOMATOES STUFFED WITH
COTTAGE CHEESE AND TUNA

Serves 4

Metric/Imperial		American
4	beefsteak tomatoes, halved	4
	salt	
150g/5oz	canned tuna in oil, drained and flaked	¾ cup
1	anchovy fillet, chopped	1
1 tsp	capers, chopped	1 tsp
150g/5oz	cottage cheese	4 tbsp
	bunch of fresh parsley, chopped	

1. Remove the seeds and most of pulp from the tomatoes. Discard the seeds and reserve the pulp. Season the tomatoes with a little salt.
2. In a mixing bowl combine the tuna, anchovy, capers, reserved tomato pulp, cottage cheese and most of the parsley.
3. Stuff the tomatoes with the mixture and sprinkle with the remaining parsley.

Note

This can be served with a mixed green salad to make a main course.

CREAM CHEESE, CELERY AND ANCHOVY CIABATTA ROLLS

Makes 2

Metric/Imperial		*American*
10	anchovy fillets in oil, drained and chopped	10
50g/2oz	cream cheese or Quark	¼ cup
1	small celery stick/stalk, thinly sliced	1
	salt and freshly ground black pepper	
	butter or soya margarine	
2	ciabatta rolls (or bagels, baguette or granary rolls)	2
	finely shredded crisp lettuce	

1. Mix together all the filling ingredients, except the lettuce.
2. Butter the rolls and spread the mixture on both halves of the rolls. Fill with the lettuce.

PROVENÇAL PAN BAGNA

Makes 4

Metric/Imperial		*American*
6 tbsp	extra virgin olive oil	6 tbsp
3 tbsp	red wine vinegar	3 tbsp
1	garlic clove, crushed	1
4	ciabatta rolls or French bread rolls, cut in half	4
8–12	anchovy fillets, drained and roughly chopped	8–12
6–8	basil leaves, roughly chopped	6–8
1	large beefsteak tomato, finely sliced	1
1	large red onion, finely sliced	1
16–20	stoned/pitted black olives, chopped	16–20
	salt and freshly ground black pepper	

1. Mix the oil, vinegar and garlic together. Trickle the mixture over the cut sides of the rolls.
2. Arrange the filling in layers on one side of the rolls. Start with the anchovies, then the basil, tomato, onion and olives. Season with salt and pepper.
3. Wrap each roll in waxed or greaseproof paper, then leave for at least 1 hour before eating to allow the dressing to be absorbed by the bread.

EGGS BENEDICT

Serves 2

Metric/Imperial		American
4 slices	wholemeal bread	4 slices
2	eggs	2
150ml/¼ pint	hollandaise sauce	⅔ cup
	butter or soya margarine	
4 thin slices	ham	4 thin slices
	parsley sprigs, to garnish	

1. Toast the bread on both sides.
2. Poach the eggs in a poacher and gently heat the sauce.
3. Lightly butter the toast, add a folded slice of ham, and top with the hot poached eggs.
4. Coat with the sauce and serve, garnished with parsley sprigs.

BAKED POTATOES

$\boxed{V}$ $\boxed{Ve}$

Metric/Imperial		*American*
1	large potato per serving (preferably King Edwards)	1

1. Prick the potatoes all over with a fork.
2. Bake in a preheated oven at 200°C/400°F/gas mark 6 for 1–2 hours depending on the size of potatoes.

Fillings
Choose from the following:

- Bacon, cooked until crisp and cut into small pieces
- Grated Cheddar cheese
- Smoked tofu, thinly sliced
- Butter
- Baked beans (low sugar)
- Fried sliced onions
- Garlic mayonnaise

SARDINE, EGG AND WATERCRESS SANDWICH

Makes 2 rounds

Metric/Imperial		American
4	canned sardines, drained and roughly chopped	4
1 large	egg, hardboiled and chopped	1 large
1 tbsp	mayonnaise	1 tbsp
2 tsp	lemon juice	2 tsp
	salt and freshly ground black pepper	
4 slices	wholemeal bread	4 slices
	butter or soya margarine	
handful	watercress, chopped	handful

1. Place the sardines and egg in a mixing bowl. Add the mayonnaise, lemon juice and seasoning, and mix well.
2. Butter the bread, fill with the sardine mixture, top with the watercress and sandwich together.

CHICKEN AND CELERY SANDWICH

Makes 2 rounds

Metric/Imperial		*American*
100g/4oz	cooked chicken, chopped	½ cup
2 sticks	celery, finely chopped	2 stalks
25g/1oz	spring onions, finely chopped	2 tbsp
1 tbsp	mayonnaise	1 tbsp
	salt and freshly ground black pepper	
4 slices	wholemeal bread	4 slices
	butter or soya margarine	
4	lettuce leaves, shredded	4

1. Place the chicken and celery in a mixing bowl. Mix in the spring onions, mayonnaise and seasoning.
2. Butter the bread, fill with the chicken mixture, top with the shredded lettuce and sandwich together.

V	Ve

ASPARAGUS AND CREAM CHEESE SANDWICH

Makes 2 rounds

Metric/Imperial		American
2 tsp	mayonnaise	2 tsp
1 tsp	chopped fresh marjoram or	1 tsp
¼ tsp	dried marjoram	¼ tsp
50g/2oz	cream cheese	¼ cup
	salt and freshly ground black pepper	
2	asparagus spears, cut into short lengths and lightly cooked (or drained canned asparagus)	2
4 slices	wholemeal bread	4 slices
	butter or soya margarine	
25g/1oz	Cheddar cheese, grated	¼ cup

1. Mix the mayonnaise with the marjoram and cream cheese.
2. Season with salt and pepper and stir in the asparagus.
3. Butter the bread, fill with the asparagus mixture, top with the cheese and sandwich together.

HERB AND MUSHROOM SANDWICH v ve

Makes 2 rounds

Metric/Imperial		American
2 tbsp	olive oil	2 tbsp
1 small	onion, finely chopped	1 small
175g/6oz	open-capped mushrooms, finely chopped	2¼ cups
1 tbsp	chopped fresh parsley	1 tbsp
2 tsp	lemon juice	2 tsp
25g/1oz	salted peanuts, chopped	2 tbsp
	salt and freshly ground black pepper	
4 slices	wholemeal bread	4 slices
	butter or soya margarine	
6	lettuce leaves, shredded	6

1. Heat the oil in a frying pan and cook the onion for 3–4 minutes, until nearly soft.
2. Stir in the mushrooms and continue cooking 5–6 minutes.
3. Mix in the parsley and lemon juice, bring to the boil then simmer until most of the liquid has evaporated. Stir in the peanuts.
4. Leave to go cold then season to taste.
5. Butter the bread, fill with the mushroom mixture, top with the lettuce and sandwich together.

CROQUE CAMPAGNARD

Serves 1

Metric/Imperial		*American*
1 thick slice	country bread (eg ciabatta, pain de campagne or any rustic wholemeal bread) butter	1 thick slice
1 thin slice	ham (Parma or Bayonne)	1 thin slice
25g/1oz	Gruyère cheese, grated	1/4 cup

1. Toast the bread very lightly on both sides.
2. Lightly butter the bread, cover with the ham and sprinkle over the cheese.
3. Cook under a preheated hot grill until the cheese begins to brown.
4. Serve with salt and pepper and Dijon mustard.

REUBEN'S DELI 'CROQUE MONSIEUR'

Makes 4 rounds

Metric/Imperial		American
2–3 tbsp	mayonnaise	2–3 tbsp
8 slices	rye bread	8 slices
4 thin slices	Gruyère cheese	4 thin slices
4 slices	corned beef	4 slices
1–2 tsp	chilli sauce	1–2 tsp
100g/4oz	sauerkraut, rinsed and drained	4 tbsp
50g/2oz	butter	¼ cup
2tbsp	virgin olive oil	2 tbsp

1. Spread the mayonnaise over 4 slices of the bread.
2. Cover the remaining slices with layers of cheese, corned beef, chilli sauce and sauerkraut (in that order). Close the sandwiches.
3. Heat the butter and oil in a frying pan, then cook the sandwiches on both sides until hot and golden brown.

TUNA SANDWICH WITH QUARK

Makes 2 rounds

Metric/Imperial		*American*
2 tbsp	Quark or fromage frais	2 tbsp
100g/4oz	canned tuna in oil, drained and flaked	⅔ cup
1 tbsp	capers, chopped	1 tbsp
	salt and freshly ground black pepper	
	butter or soya margarine	
4 slices	wholemeal bread	4 slices
4	lettuce leaves	4
1 small	tomato, thinly sliced	1 small
16 slices	cucumber	16 slices

1. Mix together the cheese, tuna and capers. Season to taste.
2. Butter the bread. Spread the tuna mixture over 2 slices of the bread. Place the lettuce, tomato and cucumber slices on top, then close the sandwiches.

PLOUGHMAN'S SANDWICH

Makes 4 rounds

Metric/Imperial		American
8 slices	wholemeal or granary bread	8 slices
	butter or soya margarine	
4 thin slices	mature Cheddar cheese or	4 thin
	blue stilton	slices
4	pickled gherkins, sliced	4
	lengthways	
4	tomatoes, sliced	4
4 large	pickled onions, sliced	4 large
	salt and freshly ground	
	black pepper	
8	lettuce leaves	8

1. Butter the bread. Cover 4 of the slices with the cheese, gherkins, tomato and onion slices, seasoning to taste. Top with the lettuce and close the sandwiches.
2. Serve with crisp eating apples or celery sticks.

SMOKED SALMON AND FETA CHEESE SANDWICH

Makes 2 rounds

Metric/Imperial		American
4 slices	wholemeal bread or 2 large rolls	4 slices
25g/1oz	butter or soya margarine	2 tbsp
2 slices	smoked salmon	2 slices
	handful of watercress, roughly chopped	
25g/1oz	feta cheese, crumbled	1/3 cup
4	basil leaves, shredded	4
	salt and freshly ground black pepper	

1. Spread the bread or rolls with the butter.
2. Fill with the salmon, and top with the watercress.
3. Sprinkle with the feta cheese and basil and season to taste.

TOASTED CROQUE MONSIEUR

Serves 1

Metric/Imperial		American
2 thin slices	white or wholemeal bread	2 thin slices
	butter or soya margarine	
2 thin slices	Gruyère or Cheddar cheese	2 thin slices
1 slice	ham	1 slice

1. Butter the bread on one side.
2. Cover one slice of bread with a slice of cheese, then the ham and another slice of cheese. Place the second slice of bread butter-side down on the top.
3. Toast under a preheated hot grill on both sides until golden.

TOASTED ASPARAGUS, HAM AND CHEESE SANDWICH

Makes 4 rounds

Metric/Imperial		American
8 slices	wholemeal bread	8 slices
4 thin slices	mature Cheddar cheese	4 thin slices
4 thin slices	lean ham	4 thin slices
225g/8oz	asparagus spears	½ lb
25g/1oz	butter, plus extra for spreading	2 tbsp

1. Cover 4 slices of the bread with the cheese and arrange the ham on top.
2. Sauté the asparagus in the butter over medium heat until tender. Chop finely and spread over the ham.
3. Butter the remaining bread and place on top of the asparagus, butter-side down.
4. Toast both sides under a preheated hot grill.

TOASTED EGG AND HERRING ROE SANDWICHES

Makes 4 rounds

Metric/Imperial		American
150g/6oz	fresh soft herring roes	1 cup
25g/1oz	butter	2 tbsp
4 large	eggs, beaten	4 large
2 tsp	chopped capers	2 tsp
8 slices	wholemeal bread	8 slices
	juice of ½ lemon	
	salt and freshly ground	
	black pepper	
	butter or soya margarine,	
	for spreading	

1. Sauté the roes in the butter for 2–3 minutes until set, then break them up in the pan.
2. Add the beaten eggs to the pan with the capers, stirring well until scrambled.
3. Toast the bread on one side. Cover 4 untoasted sides of the bread with the mixture, sprinkle on the lemon juice and season with salt and pepper.
4. Lightly spread the remaining bread with butter and place on top of the mixture, butter-side down. Serve immediately.

SANDWICH FILLING IDEAS
FOR CHILDREN

- Mashed banana with finely chopped nuts or crunchy peanut butter
- Very ripe avocado pear mashed with tofu
- Vegetarian cheese, mixed with grated carrot, raisins and finely grated nuts
- Hardboiled eggs, mashed with mayonnaise and mustard and cress
- Vegetarian pâté with sliced tomatoes or spring onions (finely sliced) or sliced cucumber
- Pear and apple spread with raisins or finely chopped nuts

Notes

- Wholemeal bread is more nutritious and usually more filling.
- Non-vegans can use butter, otherwise soya margarine or smooth peanut butter, vegetarian pâté in various flavours available from health-food stores.
- Pear and apple spread is available from health-food stores or supermarkets and is sugar-free.

BEAN AND TUNA SALAD

Serves 4

Metric/Imperial		American
200g/7oz	canned tuna in brine, drained and flaked	1 cup
400g/14oz	canned flageolet beans, rinsed and drained	2¼ cups
1	onion, sliced	1
2 tbsp	chopped fresh parsley	2 tbsp
	mixed salad leaves, roughly torn	

Dressing

	juice of ½ lemon	
3 tbsp	virgin olive oil	3 tbsp
	salt and freshly ground black pepper	

1. Place the beans in mixing bowl. Mix the dressing, pour over the beans and mix well.
2. Add the remaining ingredients, except the salad leaves, and gently mix with the beans.
3. Arrange the salad leaves in a serving dish and add the tuna and bean mixture.

THREE BEAN SALAD

Serves 4

Metric/Imperial		*American*
425g/15oz	canned red kidney beans, drained and rinsed	2⅓ cups
425g/15oz	canned borlotti beans, drained and rinsed	2⅓ cups
400g/14oz	canned flageolet beans, drained and rinsed	2¼ cups
1	Spanish onion, sliced	1
1	garlic clove, crushed	1
1 tbsp	coriander seeds	1 tbsp
4 tbsp	chopped fresh coriander	4 tbsp
3 tbsp	virgin olive oil	3 tbsp
	juice of 1 lime	
	salt and freshly ground black pepper	
225g/8oz	mixed salad greens or curly-leafed lettuce	½ lb

1. Combine the beans, onion and garlic in a large mixing bowl.
2. Dry-fry the coriander seeds, then crush with a pestle and mortar. Mix the crushed seeds with the fresh coriander and add to the bowl.
3. Mix the oil and lime juice, season and add to the salad. Mix well and leave to stand for at least 30 minutes, stirring occasionally.

Low Blood Sugar

4. Arrange the lettuce in a serving dish, pile the bean salad into the centre and serve.

WARM BULGAR WHEAT SALAD WITH GRILLED VEGETABLES

Serves 2

Metric/Imperial		American
50g/2oz	bulgar wheat	1/3 cup
150ml/1/4 pint	hot vegetable stock	2/3 cup
1 small	red pepper, cored, seeded and quartered	1 small
1 small	aubergine, sliced lengthways	1 small
1 small	courgette, sliced lengthways	1 small
4 large	chestnut mushrooms, halved	4 large
2 tsp	olive oil	2 tsp
2	canned artichoke hearts, halved	2
2	sun-dried tomatoes in oil, drained and chopped	2
few	stoned black olives	few
1 tbsp	balsamic vinegar or Vinaigrette Dressing (page 73)	1 tbsp
	fresh basil leaves, to garnish	

1. Soak the bulgar wheat in the stock for 30 minutes. Drain and place in an ovenproof serving dish. Cover with foil and keep warm in a preheated oven at 170°C/325°F/gas mark 3 while cooking the vegetables.

2. Lightly brush the pepper, courgettes and mushrooms with olive oil. Grill for about 10 minutes until golden

brown on both sides. After 8 minutes place the artichoke hearts on the grill and warm through. Remove from the heat and peel the peppers.

3. Remove the bulgar wheat from the oven and arrange the vegetables on top with any cooking juices from the grill pan.

4. Scatter the tomatoes, olives and vinegar over the vegetables.

5. Garnish with basil and serve at once.

NUT AND POTATO SALAD

Serves 4

Metric/Imperial		*American*
450g/1 lb	new potatoes	1 lb
225g/8oz	mixed green salad leaves	½ lb
1 small	cucumber, sliced	1 small
2–3 tbsp	chopped fresh parsley or mint mixed with spring onions	2–3 tbsp
12	radishes, sliced	12
100g/4oz	mixed nuts, coarsely chopped	¾ cup
	Vinaigrette Dressing (page 73)	
	salt and freshly ground black pepper	
100g/4oz	firm tofu or feta cheese cut into small cubes	1⅓ cups

1. Boil the potatoes until tender, then slice thickly and allow to cool.
2. Tear the salad leaves and place in a salad bowl. Add the cucumber, herb and spring onion mixture, radishes and nuts.
3. Add the potatoes and dressing, season and toss.
4. Sprinkle over the tofu or feta cheese and serve.

PASTA SALAD

Serves 4

Metric/Imperial		American
225g/8oz	pasta (eg fusilli, sedanini, pennette)	½ lb
4 tbsp	fromage frais	4 tbsp
3 tbsp	mayonnaise	3 tbsp
1 tbsp	white wine vinegar	1 tbsp
¼ tsp	mustard powder	¼ tsp
	salt and freshly ground black pepper	
12	radishes, quartered	12
2	celery sticks, finely chopped	2
100g/4oz	button mushrooms, quartered	1½ cups
1 tbsp	chopped fresh chives	1 tbsp

1. Cook the pasta as directed on the packet, drain and rinse under cold running water.
2. In a mixing bowl blend the fromage frais, mayonnaise, vinegar, mustard and salt and pepper to taste.
3. Stir in the pasta and the remaining ingredients except the chives. Sprinkle with the chives and serve.

PASTA SALAD WITH PRAWNS

Serves 4

Metric/Imperial		American
225g/8oz	cooked peeled prawns	½ lb
225g/8oz	cauliflower florets	½ lb
225g/8oz	small green pasta shapes	½ lb
	coriander or parsley	

Dressing

1 tbsp	virgin olive oil	1 tbsp
2 tsp	anchovy essence	2 tsp
2 tbsp	low-calorie mayonnaise	2 tbsp
	ground white pepper	

1. Defrost prawns (unless freshly cooked).
2. Separate cauliflower into small florets and boil briefly to blanch. To retain crispness, drain and rinse under cold water.
3. Cook pasta as instructed on packet. Drain and rinse under cold water.
4. Mix pasta, cauliflower and prawns and toss with dressing. Season to taste with pepper. Add coriander or parsley for a garnish and serve.

SALADE NIÇOISE

Serves 4

Metric/Imperial		*American*
450g/1 lb	tomatoes, quartered	1 lb
	salt	
1	garlic clove, halved	1
225g/8oz	mixed green salad leaves	½ lb
225g/8oz	small new potatoes, cooked and quartered	½ lb
4	eggs, hardboiled and quartered	4
100g/4oz	French beans, lightly cooked	1 cup
12–20	black olives	12–20
1	cucumber, sliced	1
8	anchovy fillets	8
225g/8oz	canned tuna in brine, drained and flaked	1⅓ cups
	Vinaigrette Dressing (page 73)	
	chopped fresh parsley or basil	

1. Sprinkle the tomatoes with salt, and set aside.
2. Rub a salad bowl with the cut garlic, then line the bowl with the salad leaves.
3. In a mixing bowl combine the potatoes, eggs, tomatoes, beans, olives, cucumber and anchovy.
4. Place the mixture on the salad leaves and sprinkle over the tuna.

5. Spoon over the dressing and garnish with chopped parsley or basil.

TABBOULEH (BULGAR WHEAT SALAD) $\boxed{V}$ $\boxed{V_e}$

Serves 4

Metric/Imperial		American
225g/8oz	coarse-grain bulgar wheat	1⅓ cups
1 small	onion, sliced	1 small
1	garlic clove, crushed	1
50g/2oz	fresh parsley, chopped	2 cups
	salt and freshly ground	
	black pepper	
25g/1oz	fresh mint, chopped	1 cup
4 tbsp	lemon juice	4 tbsp
4 tbsp	virgin olive oil	4 tbsp
100g/4oz	feta cheese or tofu, diced	1⅓ cups
225g/8oz	tomatoes, sliced	½ lb
1 small	cucumber, sliced	1 small
50g/2oz	stoned black olives	½ cup

1. Place the wheat in a mixing bowl, cover with cold water and leave to soak for 45–60 minutes.
2. Drain well, return to the mixing bowl and add the onion, garlic and parsley, mixing well. Season to taste.
3. Mix the mint, lemon juice and oil, and pour over the wheat mixture. Stir well and add more lemon juice or seasoning to taste.
4. Put into a large serving dish, and sprinkle over the cheese or tofu. Decorate the edge of the salad with the tomatoes, cucumber and olives.

| V | Ve |

GREEK SALAD

Serves 4

Metric/Imperial		American
700g/1½lb	beefsteak tomatoes	1½ lb
1	cucumber	1
1 small	lettuce	1 small
2	red onions, thinly sliced	2
125g/4oz	stoned/pitted black olives	1 cup
225g/8oz	feta cheese or tofu, diced	2⅔ cups

Dressing

3 tbsp	lemon juice	3 tbsp
9 tbsp	virgin olive oil	9 tbsp
3 tbsp	fresh coriander, chopped	3 tbsp
½ tsp	fructose	¼ tsp
	salt and freshly ground black pepper	

1. Chop the tomatoes and cucumber into bite-size chunks.
2. Tear the lettuce leaves into small pieces and place in a large salad bowl.
3. Mix the dressing ingredients well.
4. Add the tomatoes, cucumber, onions and olives to the bowl, and toss well. Pour on the dressing and toss again.
5. Sprinkle over the cheese or tofu and serve.

COUNTRY SALAD

Serves 4

Metric/Imperial		*American*
225g/8oz	asparagus	½ lb
25g/1oz	butter	2 tbsp
350g/12oz	new potatoes, boiled and cooled	¾ lb
2	eggs, hardboiled and cooled	2
1	avocado	1
50g/2oz	stoned/pitted black olives	½ cup
1 large	courgette, sliced	1 large
1 small	red onion, sliced	1 small
3 tbsp	capers	3 tbsp
	salt and freshly ground black pepper	
	Vinaigrette Dressing (page 73)	

1. Steam the asparagus or lightly sauté in the butter until tender. Cut into bite-size chunks.
2. Cut the potatoes and eggs into large slices. Peel and stone the avocado and cut into chunks.
3. Mix the ingredients together in a large serving bowl, adding dressing to taste.

SALADE LYONNAISE

Serves 4

Metric/Imperial		American
225g/8oz	mixed green salad leaves	½ lb
2 slices	granary or wholegrain bread	2 slices
2	garlic cloves, halved	2
8 rashers	streaky bacon, rinded	8 slices
	drained canned anchovies, sardines, herrings, cooked chicken liver, chopped (optional)	
4	eggs	4

1. Tear the salad leaves into bite-size pieces, and arrange in 4 individual salad bowls.
2. Toast the bread, gently rub with garlic on both sides, then cut into 2.5 cm/1 inch cubes.
3. Grill the bacon until crisp and cut into 2.5 x 5 cm/1 x 2 inch strips.
4. Add the croutons and bacon to the salad, with any of the optional ingredients, if using. Add a dressing to taste and toss.
5. Lightly poach the eggs (firm whites, runny yolks), place one on each salad and serve immediately.

VINAIGRETTE DRESSING

$\boxed{V}$ $\boxed{Ve}$

Metric/Imperial		American
3 tbsp	virgin olive oil	3 tbsp
1 tbsp	lemon juice or white wine vinegar	1 tbsp
	salt and freshly ground black pepper	
pinch	mustard powder	pinch
½ tsp	fructose	½ tsp

1. Put all the ingredients into a screw-top jar and shake vigorously.
2. Use immediately or keep chilled.

Soups, Main Meals and Desserts

The main meal of the day does not present too much of a challenge in a diet for low blood sugar. There are available a huge variety of animal and plant protein foods which can be complemented by fresh vegetables or a salad.

The recipes here include a selection of protein-rich meals, including vegan and vegetarian. Also ideas for stocks and soups and fruit-based desserts. Good quality cheese and protein biscuits (see the chapter on Between-meal Snacks) make an ideal conclusion to a meal and increase the protein component.

PARSNIP AND SESAME SOUP

$\boxed{V}$ $\boxed{Ve}$

Serves 4–6

Metric/Imperial		American
25g/1oz	soya margarine	2 tbsp
1 tbsp	oil	1 tbsp
1 large	onion, roughly chopped	1 large
450g/1 lb	parsnips, roughly chopped	1 lb
1 tsp	dried rosemary	1 tsp
600ml/1 pint	water	2½ cups
1	bay leaf	1
50g/2oz	cashew nuts, ground	½ cup
50g/2oz	sesame seeds, ground	½ cup
600ml/1 pint	soya milk	2½ cups
300ml/½ pint	apple juice	1⅓ cups
	salt and freshly ground black pepper	
1–2 tsp	sesame seeds, toasted	1–2 tsp

1. Heat the margarine and oil in a large saucepan and fry the onion for 3–4 minutes until soft but not browned.
2. Stir in the parsnips and rosemary, cover and cook for 4–5 minutes. Add the water and bay leaf, bring to the boil, cover and simmer for 25–30 minutes.
3. Remove the bay leaf, and stir in the cashew nuts, ground sesame seeds, soya milk and apple juice.
4. Liquidize in a blender or food processor until smooth and creamy (add more apple juice or water if a thinner consistency is desired).

5. To serve, reheat stirring occasionally. Do not allow to boil.
6. Season to taste and serve garnished with the whole sesame seeds.

RED LENTIL, TOMATO AND BASIL SOUP

V | Ve

Serves 4

Metric/Imperial		American
2 tbsp	sunflower oil	2 tbsp
1 large	onion, sliced	1 large
1 large	garlic clove, crushed	1 large
1	bay leaf	1
400g/14oz	canned chopped tomatoes	2 cups
pinch	dried basil	pinch
1 stick	celery, finely chopped	1 stalk
175g/6oz	split red lentils	1 cup
1.4 litres/ 2½ pints	vegetable stock	6⅓ cups
	salt and freshly ground black pepper	
	fresh basil	

1. Heat the oil in a large saucepan and fry the garlic and onion until soft but not browned.
2. Add the bay leaf, tomatoes and dried basil and cook for 2 minutes.
3. Stir in the celery, lentils and stock. Bring to the boil and continue cooking over a high heat for 15 minutes.
4. Lower the heat and simmer for 20–30 minutes until the lentils are tender.
5. Season to taste and serve garnished with fresh basil.

v **Ve**

Serves 6

Metric/Imperial		*American*
350g/12oz	dried white haricot beans, soaked overnight, drained	¾ lb
1.7 litres/ 3 pints	water	7½ cups
25g/1oz	soya margarine	2 tbsp
2 tbsp	olive oil	2 tbsp
3	garlic cloves, crushed	3
225g/8oz	onions, chopped	1⅓ cups
225g/8oz	French beans, chopped	2 cups
1.1 litres/ 2 pints	Celery Stock (page 81)	5 cups
	salt and freshly ground black pepper	

1. Put the beans and water in a large saucepan, bring to the boil, then cover and simmer for about 2 hours or until tender.
2. Heat the margarine and oil in a pan, add the garlic, onions and French beans. Cook gently for a few minutes then gradually add the stock. Cover and simmer for 20 minutes.
3. Put half the haricot beans and liquid into a blender, liquidize until smooth and pour into a saucepan.
4. Mix in the remaining beans and liquid, and add the vegetables and their stock.
5. Reheat, stirring gently, season and serve.

Low Blood Sugar

CHILLED AVOCADO SOUP

V | *Ve*

Serves 4

Metric/Imperial		American
2 large	ripe avocados	2 large
	juice and grated zest of 1 lemon	
1	garlic clove, crushed	1
	salt and freshly ground black pepper	
1.4 litres/ 2½ pints	unsweetened soya milk	6⅓ cups

1. Peel and stone the avocados and cut the flesh into chunks.
2. Put the chunks in a blender with the lemon juice and zest, garlic and seasoning.
3. Liquidize, then gradually add the milk to make a smooth thin purée.
4. Chill for at least 1 hour before serving.

VEGETABLE STOCK

Makes 1 litre/1¾ pints

Metric/Imperial		*American*
about 225g/8oz	mixed green vegetable leaves (eg cabbage, spinach, Brussels sprouts, cauliflower), chopped	½ lb
1 large	onion, chopped	1 large
1 large	carrot, chopped	1 large
1 litre/1¾ pints	water	4½ cups
	salt and freshly ground black pepper	

1. Place all the ingredients in a large saucepan, bring to the boil then cover and simmer for 30 minutes.
2. Liquidize all the ingredients in a blender, then cool and strain.
3. Keeps for up to 2 weeks in screw-top bottles in the fridge.

Note

The outer leaves of vegetables are the most flavoursome and nutritious.

CELERY STOCK

makes 1 litre/1¾ pints

Metric/Imperial		American
1	celery head, chopped	1
2	onions, chopped	2
1 litre/1¾ pints	water	4½ cups
	various flavourings (eg 2–3 bay leaves, 2 cloves garlic, sliced or 2–3 parsley stalks)	
	salt and freshly ground black pepper	

1. Place all the ingredients in a saucepan, bring to the boil then cover and simmer for at least 45 minutes.
2. Crush the vegetables with a potato masher. Allow to cool, then strain.
3. Keeps for up to 2 weeks in screw-top bottles in the fridge.

CHICKEN OR TURKEY STOCK

Metric/Imperial		American
1.4kg/3 lb	cooked chicken or turkey carcass (including neck, skin, wings, etc)	3 lb
about 1.7 litres/ 3 pints	cold water	7½ cups
1	onion, quartered	1
1	celery stick/stalk with leaves	1
1	carrot, sliced	1
	salt to taste	
1	bay leaf	1
1	bouquet garni	1

1. Break up carcass, add skin and meat.
2. Add enough cold water to cover and the remaining ingredients.
3. Bring to the boil, cover and simmer for about 2 hours.
4. Remove from the heat, strain, cool and refrigerate.
5. When cold, remove all hardened fat from the surface.
6. Use within 2–3 days or freeze for future use.

CHICK PEA AND MUSHROOM CURRY $\boxed{v}$

Serves 4

Metric/Imperial		American
3 tbsp	vegetable oil	3 tbsp
1 small	onion, chopped	1 small
2	garlic cloves, chopped	2
2 tsp	fresh ginger root, chopped	2 tsp
1 large	tomato, peeled and chopped	1 large
125ml/4fl oz	vegetable stock	½ cup
400g/14oz	canned chick peas, rinsed and drained	2¼ cups
1 tbsp	mild curry powder	1 tbsp
1 tsp	ground coriander	1 tsp
200g/8oz	rice (optional)	1 cup
225g/8oz	button mushrooms, quartered	3 cups
40	cashew nuts	40
4 tbsp	Greek yogurt	4 tbsp
2 tbsp	chopped fresh coriander (optional)	2 tbsp

1. Heat 2 tablespoons of the oil in a pan, and fry the onion, garlic and ginger for 5 minutes. Purée in a food processor with the tomato and stock until smooth.
2. Return to the pan and add the chick peas, curry powder and ground coriander.
3. Bring to the boil, cover and simmer for 20 minutes.
4. If required, cook the rice according to the packet instructions.
5. Heat the remaining oil, fry the mushrooms and nuts

Soups, Main Meals and Desserts

for 3 minutes then add to the chick pea mixture.
6. Simmer for 5 minutes, stir in the yogurt and coriander, heat through and serve with rice, if desired.

FIELD MUSHROOMS WITH ROAST TOFU AND SHALLOT STUFFING

Serves 6

Metric/Imperial		American
4 tbsp	olive oil	4 tbsp
2	garlic cloves	2
pinch	chilli powder	pinch
	salt and freshly ground black pepper	
6	giant field mushrooms, peeled	6

Marinade

150ml/¼ pint	soy sauce (good quality sauce, no sugar)	⅔ cup
150ml/¼ pint	red wine	⅔ cup
2	garlic cloves, crushed	2
1 tsp	fresh ginger root, finely chopped	1 tsp

Stuffing

350g/12oz	firm tofu, cut into 32 cubes	¾ lb
2 tbsp	sesame oil	2 tbsp
225g/8oz	shallots, quartered	½ lb
2 tbsp	olive oil	2 tbsp
	flat-leaf parsley, to garnish	

1. Mix the marinade ingredients together.

2. To make the stuffing, place the tofu in a dish and pour over the marinade. Cover and refrigerate for at least 2 hours or overnight.
3. Drain off the marinade and set aside for the sauce.
4. Gently turn the tofu cubes in the sesame oil to coat. Toss the shallots in the olive oil. Season well.
5. Arrange the shallots and tofu on a baking sheet and roast in a preheated oven at 220°C/425°F/gas mark 7 for 30 minutes.
6. Put the olive oil, garlic, chilli and seasoning in a blender and process until blended.
7. Brush the mushrooms on both sides with the oil and garlic mixture, place on an oiled baking sheet and bake until they begin to give off their juices.
8. Transfer the mushrooms to a baking dish and divide the roast shallot and tofu mixture equally between them.
9. Return to the oven and cook for 20 minutes until hot.
10. To serve, pour over the reserved marinade and garnish with parsley.

WILD MUSHROOM RISOTTO

Serves 4

Metric/Imperial		*American*
25g/1oz	dried porcini mushrooms	1/3 cup
125ml/4fl oz	boiling water	1/2 cup
2 tbsp	olive oil	2 tbsp
1 small	onion, finely chopped	1 small
350g/12oz	button mushrooms, halved if large	6 cups
350g/12oz	arborio rice	1½ cups
1.1 litres/ 2 pints	Vegetable Stock (page 80)	5 cups
15g/½oz	butter	1 tbsp
50g/2oz	Parmesan cheese or vegetarian Parmesan, grated salt and freshly ground black pepper	1/2 cup

1. Soak the porcini mushrooms in the boiling water for 15 minutes. Drain and reserve the liquid, and chop the mushrooms.
2. Heat the oil in a large frying pan, add the onion and cook for 5 minutes until golden.
3. Add the button mushrooms and chopped porcini and cook over a medium heat for 3–5 minutes.
4. Add the rice and cook, stirring, for 1 minute.
5. Add 150ml/¼ pint/²/3 cup of the stock and cook, stirring frequently, until all stock has been absorbed.

6. Gradually add the remaining stock and reserved porcini liquid until all the liquid has been absorbed.
7. Continue to cook, stirring, for 30 minutes or until the rice is tender with a cruncy middle – 'al dente'.
8. Remove the pan from the heat, stir in the butter and cheese, season to taste and serve at once with a crisp salad of mixed leaves.

BUCKWHEAT AND VEGETABLE PIE

$\boxed{V}$

Serves 3–4

Metric/Imperial		American
50g/2oz	whole green lentils	1/3 cup
1 tbsp	tomato purée	1 tbsp
25g/1oz	soya margarine	2 tbsp
175g/6oz	roasted buckwheat	1 cup
	salt and freshly ground black pepper	
2 tsp	oil	2 tsp
1 large	onion, chopped	1 large
1	green or red pepper, seeded and chopped	1
225g/8oz	mushrooms, sliced	3 cups
1	garlic clove, crushed	1
1 heaped tsp	dried oregano	1 heaped tsp
400g/14oz	canned tomatoes	2 cups
40g/1½oz	vegetarian cheese, grated	1/3 cup
25g/1oz	wholemeal breadcrumbs	1/2 cup
	cayenne pepper	
	salt and freshly ground black pepper	

1. Put the lentils in a pan with 125ml/4fl oz/½ cup of water and simmer gently for 20–30 minutes or until tender.
2. Meanwhile, mix the tomato purée with 600ml/1 pint/ 2½ cups boiling water.

3. Melt the margarine in a saucepan, add the buckwheat and stir well until the margarine has been fully absorbed.

4. Gradually pour in the tomato liquid and bring to a gentle simmer. Stir well, add a little salt, then cover and cook gently for 10 minutes.

5. Heat the oil in a frying pan, add the onion and pepper and cook for 5 minutes without browning.

6. Add the mushrooms and cook for a further 5 minutes.

7. Stir in the garlic, oregano, tomatoes and salt and pepper. Simmer gently for 10–15 minutes until some of the liquid reduces.

8. Stir in the cooked buckwheat and lentils then transfer to a lightly greased 1.4 litres/2½ pint/6¼ cup ovenproof pie dish.

9. Scatter over the grated cheese and breadcrumbs and sprinkle with cayenne pepper.

10. Bake in a preheated oven at 190°C/375°F/gas mark 5 for 20–30 minutes until golden and bubbling.

OMELETTES

Serves 1

Metric/Imperial		American
2	eggs	2
1 tbsp	water or milk	1 tbsp
	salt and freshly ground black pepper	
knob of	butter or margarine	knob of

1. Break the eggs into a mixing bowl, season and whisk gently. Stir in the water or milk.
2. Heat an omelette pan or non-stick frying pan over a gently heat. When hot add the knob of butter or margarine and heat until foaming but not brown.
3. Add the egg mixture. Stir gently with a fork or wooden spatula, drawing the mixture away from the sides of the pan to the centre as it sets. Let the liquid egg in the centre run to the sides.
4. When the eggs have set, stop stirring and cook for a further 30 seconds to 1 minute until the omelette is golden brown underneath and still creamy on top. Do not overcook or it will be tough.
5. If making a filled omelette, add the filling at this point. Tilt the pan away from you slightly and use a palette knife to fold over a third of the omelette to the centre of the pan, then fold over the opposite third.
6. Slide the omelette out onto a warm plate, letting it flip over so the folded sides are underneath.
7. Serve at once.

Soups, Main Meals and Desserts

Omelette Fillings

- Smoked tofu
  Use 25–50g/1–2oz/⅓–⅔ cup finely sliced smoked tofu.
  Spread down the centre of the omelette before folding.

- Fines herbs
  Use 1 teaspoon mixed dried herbs or 2 teaspoons
  finely chopped fresh herbs. Add to the egg mixture
  before cooking.

- Tomatoes
  Peel and chop 1–2 tomatoes, place in the centre of the
  omelette before folding.

- Mushrooms
  Use 50g/2oz/¾ cup sliced mushrooms. Cook in a
  separate pan in soya margarine or butter for 5–6 minutes,
  then place in the centre of the omelette before folding.

- Cheese
  Use 25–50g/1–2oz/¼–½ cup grated Cheddar cheese.
  Add half to the omelette mixture before cooking,
  sprinkle the remainder over the finished omelette.

- Bacon
  Fry 2 rashers of lean bacon, cut into small pieces and
  place in the centre of the omelette before folding.

- Fish
  Use 25–50g/1–2oz/¼–⅓ cup flaked cooked fish. Heat
  gently with a little cheese sauce. Place in the centre of
  the omelette before folding.

- Ham
  Add 50g/2oz/⅓ cup chopped ham and 1 teaspoon of
  chopped parsley to the omelette mixture before cooking.

Serves 6

Metric/Imperial		American
2	garlic cloves, crushed	2
2	onions, thinly sliced	2
3 tbsp	olive oil	3 tbsp
¼ tsp	dried thyme or	¼ tsp
1 tsp	chopped fresh thyme	1 tsp
450g/1 lb	button mushrooms, halved	1 lb
450g/1 lb	chestnut mushrooms, thickly sliced	1 lb
50g/2oz	butter or soya margarine	¼ cup
50g/2oz	flour	½ cup
600ml/1 pint	milk	2½ cups
	salt and freshly ground black pepper	
1 tsp	freshly grated nutmeg	1 tsp
5 sheets	no-cook lasagne	5 sheets
225g/8oz	mozzarella cheese, drained and thinly sliced	½ lb
25g/1oz	Parmesan cheese, grated	¼ cup

1. Preheat oven to 200°C/400°F/gas mark 6.
2. Fry the garlic and onions in 2 tablespoons of the olive oil for 5 minutes. Add the remaining oil, and the thyme and mushrooms, and cook for 30 minutes.
3. Melt the butter in a large pan, add the flour and cook for 1 minute. Gradually add the milk and bring to the boil. Simmer for 1 minute, stirring constantly.

Soups, Main Meals and Desserts

4. Season with salt and pepper and the nutmeg. Set aside 300ml/½ pint/1⅓ cups of the sauce. Stir the remainder into the mushroom mix.
5. Spread half the mushroom mix onto the base of a 1.7 litre/3 pint/7½ cup ovenproof dish.
6. Cover with half the pasta and repeat the mushroom layer and pasta layer. Pour over the reserved sauce.
7. Cover with the cheeses and bake for 30 minutes.

LIVER AND BACON CASSEROLE

Serves 4

Metric/Imperial		American
350g/12oz	lambs' liver, thinly sliced	3/4 lb
2 tbsp	plain flour	2 tbsp
	salt and freshly ground black pepper	
2 tbsp	oil	2 tbsp
225g/8oz	onions, thinly sliced	1/2 lb
4 rashers	streaky bacon, chopped	4 slices
225g/8oz	carrots, thinly sliced	1/2 lb
300ml/1/2 pint	beef stock	1 1/3 cups

1. Preheat oven to 180°C/350°F/gas mark 4.
2. Coat the liver slices with the seasoned flour.
3. Heat the oil in a frying pan and fry the onions for 5 minutes until soft. Add the liver and fry, turning gently, until brown.
4. Transfer the liver and onions to a casserole, and add the bacon and carrots.
5. Blend in the stock then bring to the boil, stirring constantly. Season to taste.
6. Pour the mixture into the casserole, cover and cook for 1 1/2 hours.

KEDGEREE

Serves 4

Metric/Imperial		American
175g/6oz	brown rice	3/4 cup
450g/1 lb	smoked haddock fillets	1 lb
150ml/1/4 pint	skimmed milk	2/3 cup
2	eggs, hardboiled and chopped	2
100g/4oz	frozen petit pois peas	2/3 cup
	salt and freshly ground	
	black pepper	
	chopped fresh parsley,	
	to garnish	

1. Cook the rice in a saucepan of fast-boiling salted water for about 25 minutes until tender. Drain well and rinse under cold water.
2. Poach the fish in the milk for 10–15 minutes until tender. Drain, reserving the liquid.
3. Skin and bone the fish, and flake the flesh.
4. Put the fish and rice in a pan, stir in the egg, peas and a little of the fish liquor. Add the butter and season to taste.
5. Cook gently over a low heat until thoroughly heated through. Serve garnished with parsley.

STUFFED MUSHROOMS

Serves 2

Metric/Imperial		American
4 large	field mushrooms, stalks removed and chopped	4 large
50g/2oz	wholemeal breadcrumbs	1 cup
25g/1oz	walnuts, finely chopped	3 tbsp
50g/2oz	Cheddar cheese, grated	½ cup
pinch	dried mixed herbs	pinch
1 tbsp	sugar-free tomato ketchup	1 tbsp
	freshly ground black pepper	

1. Place the mushroom caps on a greased baking sheet.
2. Mix the remaining ingredients well, including the mushroom stalks.
3. Divide the mixture into four and spoon into the mushroom caps.
4. Bake for 10 minutes in a preheated oven at 190°C/375°F/gas mark 5.

MUSHROOM AND NUT BURGERS

Serves 4

Metric/Imperial		*American*
1 small	onion, finely chopped	1 small
100g/4oz	mushrooms, finely chopped	1½ cups
1 small	courgette, finely chopped	1 small
3 tbsp	sunflower oil	3 tbsp
2 tsp	yeast extract, mixed with	2 tsp
	2 tbsp boiling water	
100g/4oz	mixed nuts, finely chopped	¾ cup
50g/2oz	hazelnuts, toasted and finely	½ cup
	chopped	
100g/4oz	wholemeal breadcrumbs	2 cups
1	egg, beaten	1
	salt and freshly ground	
	black pepper	

1. Fry the onion, mushrooms and courgette in 1 tablespoon of the oil until soft but not browned. Stir in the yeast extract mixture.

2. Place the nuts in a mixing bowl and stir in the breadcrumbs.

3. Add the vegetables and beaten egg to the bowl, stirring well.

4. Season and add extra hot water if necessary to form a stiff dough-like mixture.

5. Divide into 4 large or 8 smaller patties and fry gently in the remaining oil for 4–5 minutes on each side, until well cooked.

6. Serve with salad or vegetables, and a cheese or tomato sauce.

SOYA BEAN BURGERS

Serves 4

Metric/Imperial		American
425g/15oz	canned soya beans, rinsed and drained	2⅓ cups
100g/4oz	wheatgerm	1 cup
1 small	onion, chopped	1 small
2	eggs, beaten	2
1 tbsp	soy sauce	1 tbsp
1	tomato, skinned and pulped	1

1. Mash the beans with a potato masher.
2. Combine all the ingredients in a mixing bowl.
3. Divide the mixture into four, roll into balls and flatten into burger shapes.
4. Place on a greased baking sheet and bake in a preheated oven at 190°C/350°F/gas mark 4 for 25 minutes.
5. Turn the burgers over, bake for a further 15 minutes and serve.

REAL HAMBURGERS

Serves 2

Metric/Imperial		*American*
225g/8oz	minced beef	½ lb
	salt and freshly ground	
	black pepper	
25g/1oz	butter	2 tbsp
1 tbsp	groundnut oil	1 tbsp

1. Season the beef. Divide into two portions, form into balls and flatten into burger shapes. Do not handle heavily.
2. Heat the butter and fry the burgers until crisp on both sides, allowing 3–4 minutes for rare done. Cut open and check before eating.
3. Serve with either a tossed mixed salad or stir-fried vegetables.

Variations

- Add 2 teaspoons Dijon mustard and 1 teaspoon Worcestershire sauce to the mix.
- Add 2 tablespoons chopped fresh parsley and 2 tablespoons grated mature cheese to the mix.

v | CHICK PEA AND SPINACH TORTILLA

Serves 2

Metric/Imperial		*American*
1 tbsp	olive oil	1 tbsp
1	red onion, thinly sliced	1
1	garlic clove, crushed	1
1 tsp	ground tumeric	1 tsp
400g/14oz	canned chick peas, rinsed and drained	2¼ cups
225g/8oz	frozen leaf spinach, thawed and squeezed dry	1 cup
4	eggs, beaten salt and freshly ground black pepper	4

1. Heat the oil in a frying pan and fry the onion, garlic and tumeric for 5 minutes until soft.
2. Add the chick peas and spinach and stir well.
3. Season the eggs, stir into the pan, and cook gently for 8–10 minutes until almost set.
4. Put under a preheated grill for 2–3 minutes until set and lightly browned on top.
5. Cut into wedges and serve immediately, or allow to cool and serve cold with a crisp green salad.

LENTIL LASAGNE

Serves 2

Metric/Imperial		American
2 tsp	olive oil	2 tsp
1 small	onion, chopped	1 small
1	garlic clove, crushed	1
1 small	carrot, diced	1 small
75g/3oz	green lentils	½ cup
1 tbsp	tomato purée	1 tbsp
1 tbsp	chopped fresh parsley	⅔ cup
150ml/¼ pint	water	
	salt and freshly ground black pepper	
3 sheets	fresh lasagne	3 sheets
75g/3oz	vegetarian Cheddar cheese, grated	¾ cup

1. Heat the oil in a frying pan, add the onion and garlic and fry for 2–3 minutes. Add the carrot, cover and cook gently for 3–4 minutes.
2. Stir in the lentils, tomato purée, parsley and water, then cover and cook for 25–30 minutes until the lentils are tender, checking occasionally.
3. Uncover and cook for 3–4 minutes to thicken the mixture. Season to taste.
4. Place a layer of pasta in the base of a shallow oven-proof dish. Top with half the lentil mixture, and sprinkle with half the cheese.

5. Repeat another layer and finish with a sprinkling of cheese.
6. Bake the lasagne in a preheated oven at 190°C/375°F/gas mark 5 for 20–25 minutes or until cooked and golden.

Note

Dried lasagne can be used, but pre-cook before use as directed on the packet.

LAMB FILLET WITH LEEKS
AND LENTILS

Serves 4

Metric/Imperial		American
450g/1 lb	lamb neck fillet, cut into 2.5 cm/1 inch slices	1 lb
1 small	onion, finely chopped	1 small
125ml/4fl oz	fresh orange juice	½ cup
	salt and freshly ground black pepper	
1 tbsp	oil	1 tbsp
450g/1 lb	small leeks, cut into 1 cm/½ inch slices	1 lb
100g/4oz	split red lentils	½ cup
1 tsp	paprika	1 tsp
300ml/½ pint	lamb stock	1⅓ cups

1. Place the lamb in a glass or ceramic dish, and sprinkle over the onion.
2. Pour on the orange juice and season with pepper. Cover and chill for 12 hours, turning the meat once in the marinade.
3. Remove the meat from the marinade and pat dry on kitchen paper. Reserve the marinade.
4. Heat the oil in a frying pan and seal the meat on both sides. Remove from the pan and drain on kitchen paper.

5. Add the leeks, lentils and paprika to the pan and stir over a moderate heat for 1 minute. Place the meat back on the lentils. Pour in the reserved marinade and the stock and bring gently to the boil.
6. Cover and simmer gently for 20 minutes, then season to taste.
7. Serve with boiled new potatoes (skins left on).

SPANISH OMELETTE

$\boxed{V}$

Serves 2

Metric/Imperial		American
4	eggs, beaten	4
2	onions, finely chopped	2
1–2	garlic cloves, crushed	1–2
450g/1 lb	firm tomatoes, skinned, seeded and chopped	1 lb
2	green peppers, seeded and cut into fine strips	2
15g/½oz	butter	1 tbsp
½ tbsp	olive oil	½ tbsp
½ tsp	chopped fresh basil salt and freshly ground black pepper	½ tsp

1. Heat the butter and olive oil in a heavy frying pan, add the onions and cook gently for 10–15 minutes without browning.
2. Stir in the garlic, tomatoes, peppers, basil and seasoning.
3. Cook uncovered for 20 minutes, stirring occasionally.
4. Pour the eggs into the pan, and using a wooden spoon stir as for scrambled eggs.
5. As soon as the mixture starts to thicken, take off the heat and continue stirring until the mixture sets. Do not allow to overcook.
6. Serve with sliced chorizo sausage or Bayonne ham, if liked.

Soups, Main Meals and Desserts

ITALIAN RABBIT

Serves 6

Metric/Imperial		American
40g/1½oz	butter	3 tbsp
1	rabbit, jointed	1
1	onion, finely chopped	1
6	shallots, finely chopped	6
1	carrot, finely chopped	1
3	garlic cloves, finely chopped	3
300ml/½ pint	white wine	1⅓ cups
300ml/½ pint	beef stock	1⅓ cups
1	bouquet garni	1
2 tbsp	tomato purée	2 tbsp
225g/8oz	mushrooms, quartered	3 cups
2 tbsp	cornflour	2 tbsp

1. Melt the butter in a casserole, add the rabbit, bacon, onion, shallots, carrot and garlic and sauté until the rabbit is browned all over.
2. Add the wine and beef stock to cover, bouquet garni and seasoning.
3. Cover and simmer for 1 hour.
4. Stir in the tomato purée and mushrooms, and cook for a further 30 minutes.
5. Just before serving, mix the cornflour with a little water, stir into the casserole and bring to the boil to thicken the mixture.
6. Serve with cooked rice or pasta.

MAGGIE'S FISH PIE

Serves 4

Metric/Imperial		American
700g/1½ lb	cod fillet (or mixed white fish fillets and shelled cooked prawns)	1½ lb
1	bay leaf	1
	salt and freshly ground black pepper	
about 600ml/1 pint	water	about 2½ cups
50g/2oz	soya margarine	¼ cup
40g/1½oz	plain flour	¼ cup
300ml/½ pint	soya milk	1⅓ cups
2 tbsp	chopped fresh parsley	2 tbsp
2	eggs, hardboiled and roughly chopped	2

Topping

450g/1 lb	potatoes, boiled and mashed with a little butter	1 lb
40g/1½oz	Cheddar cheese, grated	⅓ cup

1. Place the cod (or other white fish) in a large pan, add the bay leaf and salt and pepper, and enough water to cover. Poach gently for about 15 minutes.
2. Remove the fish with a slotted spoon, strain and reserve the cooking liquid. Remove and discard the skin and bones from the fish and flake the flesh.

3. In a small pan melt the margarine, add the flour and stir together. Cook well for 2 minutes stirring constantly.
4. Gradually blend in the milk, about 150ml/¼ pint/⅔ cup of the reserved fish liquor, and the prawns (if using).
5. Bring to the boil and simmer for 2 minutes, stirring until a smooth sauce has formed.
6. Add the flaked fish, parsley and hardboiled eggs. Season to taste.
7. Pour the mixture into a pie dish, cover with the mashed potato and sprinkle over the cheese.
8. Place under a preheated hot grill until golden brown and crisp.

MAGGIE'S CHICKEN CACCIATORA

Serves 4

Metric/Imperial		American
25g/1oz	butter	2 tbsp
½ tbsp	oil	½ tbsp
2 sticks	celery, sliced	2 stalks
1	onion, chopped	1
225g/8oz	tomatoes, skinned and chopped, or	½ lb
400g/14oz	canned chopped tomatoes	2 cups
1	garlic clove, crushed	1
	salt and freshly ground black pepper	
pinch	cayenne	pinch
350g/12oz	cooked chicken, diced	¾ lb
75g/3oz	long-grain rice	¾ cup
600ml/1 pint	chicken stock	2½ cups
	freshly grated Parmesan cheese, to taste	

1. Fry the vegetables gently in the oil and butter until nearly tender. Season well.
2. Add the chicken and allow to heat through.
3. Meanwhile, cook the rice in the stock for about 20 minutes or until the rice is tender and most of the liquid absorbed.
4. Place the rice on a warmed serving dish, top with the chicken mixture and sprinkle over Parmesan cheese.

APPLE AND HAZELNUT YOGURT

Serves 4

Metric/Imperial		*American*
125ml/4fl oz	natural unsweetened apple juice	1/2 cup
450g/1 lb	apples, cored and sliced	1 lb
450ml/3/4 pint	natural yogurt	13/4 cups
1 tsp	grated lemon zest	1 tsp
50g/2oz	hazelnuts, toasted and chopped	1/2 cup

1. Place the apple juice and apple slices in a pan, bring to the boil and simmer gently for 5–10 minutes.
2. Put into a blender, add the yogurt and blend together.
3. Pour the mixture into a serving dish and stir in the lemon zest and hazelnuts.
4. Chill well before serving.

DATE AND BANANA ICE-CREAM

$\boxed{V}$ $\boxed{Ve}$

Serves 4

Metric/Imperial		*American*
225g/8oz	dried dates, stoned	½ lb
600ml/1 pint	water	2½ cups
1	vanilla pod	1
6 tbsp	vegetable oil	6 tbsp
100g/4oz	soya milk powder	1 cup
3	bananas, peeled and sliced	3

1. Place the dates, water and vanilla pod in a pan, bring to the boil, then cover and simmer for 15–20 minutes until the dates are very soft.
2. Allow to cool a little and remove the vanilla pod.
3. Pour into a blender and liquidize with the remaining ingredients until smooth and creamy.
4. Either freeze in an ice-cream maker or transfer to a plastic container and freeze for at least 2–3 hours before serving.

BAKED STUFFED PEACHES

Serves 4

Metric/Imperial		American
4 large	ripe peaches	4 large
75g/3oz	ground almonds	¾ cup
3 tbsp	fresh orange juice	3 tbsp
150ml/5fl oz	natural unsweetened orange juice	⅔ cup

1. Slice the top off each peach and carefully remove the stone.
2. Mix the almonds and fresh orange juice to a stiff mixture, then stuff the peaches and replace the tops.
3. Stand the peaches in an ovenproof dish and pour in the natural unsweetened orange juice.
4. Bake in a preheated oven at 190°C/375°F/gas mark 5 for 30 minutes until tender.
5. Leave to cool for 5–10 minutes. Place in individual serving dishes and spoon over a little of the cooking juices.

DRIED FRUIT COMPOTE

| v | ve |

Serves 4

Metric/Imperial		*American*
50g/2oz	dried pears	1/3 cup
50g/2oz	dried prunes	1/3 cup
50g/2oz	dried apricots	1/3 cup
50g/2oz	dried peaches	1/3 cup
50g/2oz	dried apples	1/3 cup
3	cloves	3
1	cinnamon stick/stalk	1
	grated zest of 1 large orange	

1. Place the dried fruit in a saucepan, add enough water to cover and bring to the boil.
2. Remove from the heat, then cover and leave to stand for 1 hour.
3. Drain the fruit, reserving 450ml/15fl oz/2 cups of the juice. Heat the juice with the cloves, cinnamon stick and fruit until boiling.
4. Simmer gently for 30 minutes until the fruit is soft. Leave to cool.
5. Serve chilled, sprinkled with the orange zest.

⟨ν⟩ PEARS BAKED WITH SESAME SEEDS

Serves 4

Metric/Imperial		*American*
4	pears	4
25–50g/1–2oz	butter, melted	2 tbsp–¼ cup
25–50g/1–2oz	sesame seeds	¼–⅓ cup
pinch	grated nutmeg	pinch
150ml/5fl oz	natural unsweetened apple juice	⅔ cup

1. Cut the pears in half and remove the cores. Either peel, or leave the skins on.
2. Place in an ovenproof dish, brush with the melted butter, scatter over the sesame seeds and sprinkle with the nutmeg.
3. Pour the apple juice into the dish and bake in a preheated oven at 190°C/375°F/gas mark 5 for 30–35 minutes until tender.

BANANA BREAD PUDDING

V	Ve

Serves 4

Metric/Imperial		*American*
100g/4oz	fresh breadcrumbs	2 cups
1 large	banana, thinly sliced	1 large
75g/3oz	mixed dried fruit	½ cup
25g/1oz	soya margarine	2 tbsp
300ml/½ pint	soya milk	1⅓ cups
½ tsp	almond essence	½ tsp
50g/2oz	flaked almonds	½ cup

1. Grease a pie dish, cover the bottom with one-third of the breadcrumbs. Top with half the banana slices and half the dried fruit.
2. Repeat the layering, finishing with a final layer of breadcrumbs.
3. Dot the surface with the margarine.
4. Mix the milk with the almond essence, pour over the pudding and sprinkle with the flaked almonds.
5. Bake in a preheated oven at 200°C/400°F/gas mark 6 for 25–30 minutes until golden brown.

BAKED APPLES STUFFED WITH FIGS

Serves 4

Metric/Imperial		*American*
4 large	cooking apples	4 large
50g/2oz	dried figs, finely chopped	1/3 cup
50g/2oz	mixed coarsely chopped nuts	1/2 cup
25g/1oz	sunflower seeds	1/4 cup
25g/1oz	butter or soya margarine	2 tbsp
150ml/5fl oz	natural unsweetened apple juice	2/3 cup

1. Core the apples and score a slit around the middles to prevent bursting.
2. Mix the figs, nuts and sunflower seeds together, and stuff into the apples.
3. Place the apples in a shallow ovenproof dish, dot a little butter over each apple, then pour over the apple juice.
4. Bake in a preheated oven at 190°C/375°F/gas mark 5 for 30–35 minutes until soft.

BAKED APPLES STUFFED WITH PRUNES V Ve

Serves 4

Metric/Imperial		American
4 large	cooking apples	4 large
12	prunes, stoned/pitted and chopped coarsely	12
1/4 tsp	ground cinnamon	1/4 tsp
1 tbsp	slivered almonds	1 tbsp
225ml/8fl oz	natural unsweetened apple juice	1 cup

1. Core the apples and score a slit around the middles to prevent bursting.
2. Combine the prunes, cinnamon and almonds, and stuff into the apples.
3. Place the apples in a shallow ovenproof dish and pour over the apple juice.
4. Bake in a preheated oven at 190°C/375°F/gas mark 5 for 25–30 minutes until soft.

4

Between-meal Snacks and Drinks

An essential element in controlling low blood sugar is the question of meal frequency. It is often advisable to have a protein snack between meals and at bedtime, to prevent swings in the blood sugar levels.

A sit-down meal, mid-morning and mid-afternoon at school or the office is often inconvenient. The recipes in this section offer a choice of high-protein snacks and drinks that can be easily prepared and eaten on these occasions.

An electric blender is a great help with the drinks, all of which can be mixed in minutes.

PEANUT AND RAISIN COOKIES

Makes 20

Metric/Imperial		*American*
50g/2oz	soya margarine	1/4 cup
100g/4oz	raisins, minced	2/3 cup
50g/2oz	smooth peanut butter	1/2 cup
4 tbsp	water	4 tbsp
1 tsp	vanilla essence	1 tsp
1	egg	1
200g/7oz	81% wholemeal flour	1 3/4 cups
1/2 tsp	baking powder	1/4 tsp
1 tsp	bicarbonate of soda	1 tsp
a little	skimmed milk	a little
50g/2oz	salted peanuts, chopped	1/2 cup

1. Put the margarine, raisins and peanut butter in a mixing bowl and mix well.
2. Add the water, vanilla and egg, beating well.
3. Mix in the flour, baking powder and bicarbonate of soda.
4. Place teaspoons of the mixture on a baking tray, flatten each one, and brush with skimmed milk.
5. Press the chopped peanuts into each cookie, then bake in a preheated oven at 170°C/325°F/gas mark 3 for 15 minutes until golden.

DIGESTIVE BISCUITS

Makes about 25

Metric/Imperial		*American*
50g/2oz	soya flour	½ cup
150g/5oz	81% wholemeal flour (fine-milled)	1¼ cups
1 tsp	baking powder	1 tsp
½ tsp	salt	½ tsp
40g/1½oz	fine oatmeal	⅓ cup
100g/4oz	soya margarine	½ cup
50g/2oz	fructose	⅓ cup
2–3 tbsp	concentrated soya milk	2–3 tbsp

1. Sift the flour, baking powder and salt into a mixing bowl. Stir in the oatmeal.
2. Rub in the margarine until the mixture resembles breadcrumbs.
3. Mix in the fructose and enough soya milk to make a soft dough.
4. Roll out to 5 mm/¼ inch thickness and cut into biscuits using a 5.6 cm/2¼ inch cutter.
5. Place on a non-stick baking sheet, and bake in a preheated oven at 180°C/350°F/gas mark 4 for 15–20 minutes until firm and golden.
6. Transfer to a wire rack to cool.

CORNMEAL AND SESAME CRACKERS v

Makes 24

Metric/Imperial		American
25g/1oz	butter, melted, plus extra for greasing	2 tbsp
100g/4oz	quick-cook polenta	1 cup
½ tsp	salt	½ tsp
350ml/12fl oz	boiling water	1½ cups
1 tsp	sesame oil	1 tsp
25g/1oz	sesame seeds	¼ cup

1. Grease 2–3 baking sheets with a little butter.
2. Put the polenta and salt in a heatproof bowl, add the boiling water and stir vigorously until smooth.
3. Stir in the butter and sesame oil. The mixture should have the consistency of thin cream, if not add cold water as required.
4. For each cracker, spoon 1 tablespoon of mixture onto a baking sheet and spread to make a thin circle (about 4–5 per sheet). Sprinkle with sesame seeds.
5. Bake in batches in a preheated oven at 200°C/400°F/ gas mark 6 for 20–25 minutes until the edges begin to turn brown and crisp.
6. Transfer to a wire rack to cool.

CHEESE CRUNCHIES

Makes 20–25

Metric/Imperial		*American*
100g/4oz	81% wholemeal flour	1 cup
40g/1½oz	soya margarine	3 tbsp
50g/2oz	Cheddar cheese, grated	½ cup
½ tsp	mustard powder	½ tsp
1	egg yolk	1
1½ tbsp	water	1½ tbsp

1. Put the flour and margarine in a mixing bowl and mix with a fork.
2. Add the cheese and mustard, and mix well. Stir in the egg yolk and water.
3. Knead the mixture to form a stiff dough, then chill for 15 minutes.
4. Roll out the dough on a floured surface to 5 mm/½ inch thickness, and cut into 5 cm/2 inch diameter biscuits.
5. Place on a greased baking tray and bake in a preheated oven at 180C/350F/gas mark 4 for about 15 minutes. Do not allow to overcook.
6. Transfer to a wire rack to cool.

NUTTY OAT BISCUITS

$\boxed{\text{V}}$ $\boxed{\text{Ve}}$

Makes 16

Metric/Imperial		*American*
50g/2oz	ground almonds	½ cup
75g/3oz	rolled oats	¾ cup
25g/1oz	desiccated coconut	⅓ cup
25g/1oz	soya margarine	2 tbsp
2 tbsp	pear and apple spread	2 tbsp
½ tsp	vanilla essence	½ tsp

1. Combine all the ingredients in a mixing bowl and mix well.
2. Divide the mixture into 16 equal pieces, then roll each one into a ball.
3. Place the balls on a greased or non-stick baking tray, and press your thumb into the middle of each ball.
4. Bake in a preheated oven at 170°C/325°F/gas mark 3 for 10–12 minutes until golden.
5. Transfer to a wire rack to cool.

BANANA MILK

Serves 4

Metric/Imperial		American
1 small	ripe banana, sliced	1 small
1	egg	1
1 tbsp	skimmed milk powder	1 tbsp
1 tbsp	fructose	1 tbsp
1 tsp	smooth peanut butter	1 tsp
1 litre/1¾ pints	soya milk	4½ cups

1. Place the banana, egg, skimmed milk powder, fructose, and peanut butter with 300ml/½ pint/1⅓ cups of the soya milk in a blender.
2. Blend until smooth, then add the remaining soya milk.
3. Serve hot or cold.

CASHEW MILK

Serves 4

Metric/Imperial   *American*
100g/4oz   cashew nuts   1 cup
1 litre/1¾ pints water   4½ cups

1. Place the ingredients in a blender and blend for 2
   minutes.
2. Keep chilled in a sealed container.

Note

As cashew nuts are naturally sweet you should not need
to add flavourings.

SEED AND NUT MILK

Serves 3

Metric/Imperial		*American*
25g/1oz	sunflower seeds	1/4 cup
75g/3oz	blanched almonds	3/4 cup
650ml/23fl oz	water	3 cups
1 tbsp	fructose	1 tbsp
pinch	salt	pinch
150ml/5fl oz	soya milk	2/3 cup

1. Place the seeds, nuts and 300ml/1/2 pint/1 1/3 cups of the water in a blender. Allow to soak for 15–20 minutes, then blend until smooth.
2. Add the fructose, remaining water, soya milk and salt, and blend until well mixed.
3. Keep chilled in a sealed container.

HIGH PROTEIN MILK

Serves 6–8

Metric/Imperial		American
4	eggs	4
150ml/5fl oz	natural yogurt	2/3 cup
2 tbsp	soya oil	2 tbsp
1 litre/1¾ pints	water	4½ cups
225g/8oz	soya flour	2 cups
225g/8oz	skimmed milk powder	2⅔ cups

1. Place the eggs, yogurt and oil in a blender and blend until smooth.
2. Add the remaining ingredients, and blend until well mixed.
3. Keep chilled in a sealed container.

EGG AND SOYA DRINK

Serves 6–7

Metric/Imperial		American
1 tbsp	soya oil	1 tbsp
2	egg yolks	2
150ml/5fl oz	natural yogurt	⅔ cup
150ml/5fl oz	skimmed milk	⅔ cup
150ml/5fl oz	soya milk or	⅔ cup
25g/1oz	soya flour	¼ cup
150ml/5fl oz	fresh orange juice (or other fresh fruit juice)	⅔ cup
1 litre/1¾ pints	milk	4½ cups

1. Place all the ingredients with 300ml/½ pint/1⅓ cups of the milk in a blender and blend until smooth.
2. Stir in the remaining milk.
3. Keep chilled in a sealed container.

SESAME MILK

Serves 4

Metric/Imperial		American
100g/4oz	sesame seeds	3/4 cup
1.1 litres/ 2 pints	water	5 cups
	fructose to taste (optional)	

1. Place all the ingredients in a blender, blend for 2 minutes then strain well.
2. Keep chilled in a sealed container.

QUICK BREAKFAST DRINK

Serves 1

Metric/Imperial		*American*
150ml/5fl oz	natural yogurt	2/3 cup
150ml/5fl oz	fresh orange juice	2/3 cup
1 small	banana, sliced	1 small
1	egg yolk	1

1. Place all the ingredients in a blender and blend until smooth.
2. Serve very cold with ice.

QUICK PROTEIN DRINK

Serves 1

Metric/Imperial		*American*
150ml/5fl oz	soya milk	⅔ cup
1	egg	1
150ml/5fl oz	fresh orange juice	⅔ cup

1. Place all the ingredients in a blender and blend until smooth.
2. Serve chilled.

5

Pâtés, Dips, Cheeses and Chutneys

Dips, pâtés and cheeses are very versatile foods and they can be prepared for breakfast, lunch, tea, supper or snacks between meals. An electric blender is indispensible for many of these dishes.

It is very difficult to buy pickles and chutney that are sugar free, so the recipes in this chapter should prove useful.

Sugar-free tomato and brown sauces are available from some supermarkets and most health food shops.

MUSHROOM AND CASHEW NUT PÂTÉ $\boxed{V}$ $\boxed{Ve}$

Serves 8

Metric/Imperial		American
3 tbsp	vegetable oil	3 tbsp
50g/2oz	unsalted cashew nuts	½ cup
700g/1½ lb	open-cap mushrooms, chopped	1½ lb
2	garlic cloves, crushed	2
1 level tsp	dried thyme	1 level tsp
½ level tsp	cayenne pepper	½ level tsp
½ level tsp	ground allspice	½ level tsp
200g/7oz	silken tofu	1 cup
2 level tbsp	chopped fresh parsley	2 level tbsp
	salt and freshly ground black pepper	

1. Heat the oil in a heavy-based frying pan and fry the nuts for 2–3 minutes until browned. Remove from the pan and set aside to cool.
2. Add the mushrooms, garlic, thyme, cayenne and allspice to the pan. Cook, stirring constantly for 10 minutes or until the mushrooms are very soft. Allow to cool slightly.
3. Process the nuts in a food processor until finely chopped, then put into a bowl.

4. Put the tofu into the food processor and process until smooth. Add the mushroom mixture and process until finely chopped, then add the nuts and parsley.
5. Season well, adding extra cayenne and allspice if required.
6. Spoon the pâté into a serving dish, cover and chill. Remove from the fridge about 30 minutes before serving.

Note

Keeps for up to 1 week.

CHICKEN LIVER PÂTÉ

Serves 4

Metric/Imperial		*American*
25g/1oz	soya margarine	2 tbsp
1	onion, finely chopped	1
225g/8oz	chicken livers	½ lb
1 tsp	freshly grated nutmeg	1 tsp
	salt and freshly ground black pepper	
1	lemon slice, to garnish	1

1. Heat the margarine in a pan and lightly sauté the onion for 1 minute.
2. Add the chicken livers, nutmeg and seasoning and continue cooking for 5–6 minutes, stirring occasionally.
3. Leave to cool then liquidize in a blender until smooth.
4. Put the pâté in a serving dish and smooth the top. Garnish with the lemon slice and chill until required.

Note

Keeps for up to 2 days.

SMOKED MACKEREL PÂTÉ

Serves 4

Metric/Imperial		*American*
225g/8oz	smoked mackerel fillets, skinned and flaked	1⅓ cups
100g/4oz	skimmed milk soft cheese	½ cup
	lemon juice, to taste	
	salt and freshly ground black pepper	

1. Mix the ingredients together well in a mixing bowl, or process in a liquidizer until smooth.
2. Put the pâté in a serving dish and chill until required.

Note

Keeps for up to 2 days.

TOFU PÂTÉ

V | Ve

Serves 4

Metric/Imperial		American
225g/8oz	packet smoked tofu	½ lb
50g/2oz	walnut pieces, ground	½ cup
25g/1oz	wholemeal breadcrumbs	½ cup
2–3 drops	Tabasco	2–3 drops
25g/1oz	butter or soya margarine	2 tbsp
2 tsp	soy sauce (shoyu or tamari)	2 tsp
	freshly ground black pepper	

1. Place all the ingredients in a mixing bowl and mix into a smooth ball. Season to taste with pepper.
2. Spoon the pâté into a serving dish and chill until required.

Note

Keeps for up to 3 days if refrigerated.

CRUDITÉS

A selection of washed, trimmed, raw vegetables can be used with any of the following dips.

red and yellow peppers
young carrots
celery
fennel
cucumber
cauliflower or broccoli

Cut the vegetables into strips or batons. Cauliflower or broccoli can be trimmed into florets.

radishes
spring onions
cherry tomatoes

These can be left whole.

Note

Crudités can also be made from fresh fruit. Try apples, pears, nectarines, grapes, mangoes, dates, dried figs, dates and apricots. Serve with a savoury dip to give the taste buds a jolt!

GARLIC DIP

Serves 4

Metric/Imperial		American
50g/2oz	wholemeal breadcrumbs	1 cup
4 large sprigs	parsley, stalks removed	4 large sprigs
75g/3oz	ground almonds	¾ cup
3 tbsp	lemon juice	3 tbsp
2 tbsp	apple juice	2 tbsp
2 tbsp	olive oil	2 tbsp
4	garlic cloves, crushed	4
	salt and freshly ground black pepper	
150ml/¼ pint	fromage frais	⅔ cup

1. Place the breadcrumbs, parsley, almonds, lemon and apple juice, olive oil, garlic and seasoning in a food processor. Blend until a paste is formed.
2. Turn the mixture into a bowl and add the fromage frais.
3. Chill before serving. Serve fresh or within 24 hours.

HUMMUS

Serves 4

Metric/Imperial		*American*
150g/5oz	chick peas, soaked overnight	1 cup
2	garlic cloves, crushed	2
1 tsp	salt	1 tsp
	freshly ground black pepper	
6 tbsp	tahini	6 tbsp
	juice of 2 lemons	
	olive oil	

1. Drain the chick peas and put in a saucepan with enough water to cover. Bring to the boil and boil briskly for 10 minutes, then cover and simmer for 1–1½ hours until tender.
2. Drain, then rinse the peas (optional), place in a food processor and blend to a smooth paste.
3. Gradually blend in the garlic, salt, pepper, tahini and lemon juice. Add a little of the chick pea cooking water if the mixture is too thick. Season to taste.
4. Turn the mixture into a serving dish and pour a little olive oil over the surface.
5. Chill if desired, then serve immediately or within 24 hours.

SAVOURY PEANUT DIP

Serves 6–8

Metric/Imperial		American
450g/1 lb	tofu, diced	1 lb
2	lemons, juice of	2
5 tbsp	olive oil	5 tbsp
5 tbsp	peanut butter	5 tbsp
5 tbsp	soya milk	5 tbsp
3 tbsp	soy sauce	3 tbsp
1 tsp	mustard powder	1 tsp
2 tsp	grated fresh ginger root or	2 tsp
1½ tsp	dried ginger	1½ tsp
1 tsp	freshly ground black pepper	1 tsp
½ tsp	cayenne pepper	½ tsp

1. Place all the ingredients in a food processor and blend
   to a smooth cream. Add a little water if it seems too
   thick.
2. Turn into a serving dish and chill for at least 30 minutes
   before serving. Best served within 24 hours.

TOFU AND TAHINI DIP

Serves 4–6

Metric/Imperial		American
225g/8oz	tofu, diced	½ lb
2 tsp	tahini	2 tsp
1 tbsp	soy sauce	1 tbsp
1 tbsp	dry or medium sherry	1 tbsp
1–2 tbsp	chutney	1–2 tbsp
1 tbsp	apple concentrate	1 tbsp
	salt and freshly ground black pepper	
4	spring onions, chopped	4
1 tsp	sesame seeds	1 tsp

1. Blend all the ingredients except the spring onions and sesame seeds in a liquidizer.
2. Stir in the chopped onions and adjust the seasoning. Turn into a serving bowl.
3. Dry roast the sesame seeds in a heavy pan until golden brown. Allow to cool, then sprinkle over the dip.
4. Chill if desired, then serve immediately or within 24 hours.

EASY MACKEREL DIP

Serves 4

Metric/Imperial		American
75g/3oz	mackerel canned in brine	½ cup
75g/3oz	ricotta cheese	⅓ cup
25g/1oz	butter or soya margarine	2 tbsp
	juice of ½ lemon	
1 tbsp	finely chopped spring onions	1 tbsp
	freshly ground black pepper	

1. Drain the fish and remove the bones.
2. Put the fish in a blender with the remaining ingredients and blend until smooth.
3. Adjust the seasoning, turn into a serving dish and chill until required.

Note

Keeps for up to 2 days.

SEED AND NUT SOFT CHEESE

Makes 225–250g/8–9oz/¹/₂ lb

Metric/Imperial		American
50g/2oz	mixed nuts, chopped	3 tbsp
25g/1oz	sunflower seeds	¼ cup
25g/1oz	sesame seeds	¼ cup
50g/2oz	soft sunflower margarine	¼ cup
3 tbsp	sunflower oil	3 tbsp
50g/2oz	soya flour	½ cup
	chopped mixed fresh herbs or crushed garlic (optional)	

1. Spread the nuts and seeds on a baking tray and toast under a medium-hot grill for 5–7 minutes, turning occasionally, until browned.
2. Allow to cool, then grind finely.
3. Heat the margarine and oil in a pan and stir in the nut and seed mixture until evenly blended.
4. Add the flour and herbs or garlic, if using. Mix well then turn into a serving dish and keep chilled.
5. Will keep, covered, for up to 7 days.

Note

An ideal filling for jacket potatoes.

MIXED SEED SOFT CHEESE

$\boxed{V}$ $\boxed{Ve}$

Makes 275g–300g/10–11oz/³⁄₄ lb

Metric/Imperial		American
2 tbsp	sunflower seeds	2 tbsp
2 tbsp	pumpkin seeds	2 tbsp
1 tbsp	poppy seeds	1 tbsp
1 tbsp	sesame seeds	1 tbsp
1 tsp	caraway seeds	1 tsp
5 tbsp	sunflower, safflower or corn oil	5 tbsp
25g/1oz	soya flour	¼ cup
8–9 tbsp	apple juice	8–9 tbsp

1. Mix all the seeds together and grind finely.
2. Heat the oil slightly in a pan and mix in the ground seeds and flour
3. Add the apple juice slowly, beating well until a soft, creamy consistency is obtained. Turn into a serving dish and keep chilled.
4. Will keep, covered, for up to 7 days.

Note
An ideal filling for jacket potatoes.

PEGGY'S BEAN CHUTNEY

Makes 1.8–2/3 kg/4–5 lb

Metric/Imperial		American
675g/1½ lb (prepared weight)	runner beans	1½ lb
450g/1 lb (prepared weight)	chopped onions	1 lb
575ml/1pint	malt vinegar	2½ cups
1 tbsp (heaped)	dried mustard	1 tbsp
1 tbsp (heaped)	cornflour	1 tbsp
1 tbsp (heaped)	turmeric	1 tbsp
350g/12oz	fructose	¾ lb
	salt and freshly ground black pepper to taste	

1. String and slice beans and cook until tender.
2. Cook onions in 300ml/½ pint/1⅓ cups vinegar.
3. Mix the mustard, cornflour and turmeric with a little vinegar into a smooth paste.
4. Drain the beans and boil for a further 10 minutes in the remaining vinegar.
5. Add the onions, paste and fructose to the beans and boil for a further 15 minutes.
6. Add salt and pepper to taste.
7. Put into warm jars, seal and store.

PICCALILLI

V | Ve

Makes 1.8–2.3 kg/4–5 lb

Metric/Imperial		American
1 kg/2.2 lb	mixed vegetables (eg green beans, baby cucumbers, celery, cauliflower florets)	2.2 lb
875ml/1½ pints	malt vinegar	3¾ cups
2 tbsp	cornflour	2 tbsp
½ tsp	chilli powder	½ tsp
25g/1oz	mustard powder	¼ cup
3 tsp	turmeric	3 tsp
1 tsp	salt	1 tsp
150ml/¼ pint	water	⅔ cup
20–25	pickled cocktail onions	20–25
100g/4oz	fructose	⅔ cup

1. Cut the beans, cucumbers and celery into chunks.
2. Place in a pan of simmering water, add the cauliflower florets and simmer for 10 minutes. Drain well.
3. Return the vegetables to the pan, add the vinegar and bring to the boil.
4. Mix together the cornflour, chilli powder, mustard powder, turmeric and salt, and gradually stir in the water.
5. Remove the vegetables from the heat, and stir in the cornflour mixture and onions.
6. Add the fructose to taste, bring back to a gentle boil, then simmer for about 10 minutes, stirring constantly.

7. Allow to cool slightly, then spoon into warm jars, seal and store.

6

Baking

The breads in this chapter are all protein-rich, with a low fat, sugar-free and high complex carbohydrate and protein content. Ideal for the whole family, they can be used as toast for breakfast or supper or to make sandwiches for lunch.

QUICK AND EASY WHOLEMEAL BREAD (HIGH PROTEIN)

Makes 2

Metric/Imperial		*American*
300g/12oz	wholemeal flour	3 cups
100g/4oz	soya flour	1 cup
1 tsp	fructose	1 tsp
2 tsp	salt	2 tsp
25g/1oz	soya margarine	2 tbsp
7g/¼oz	sachet easy-bake yeast	½ tbsp
300ml/½ pint	tepid water	1⅓ cups

1. Put the flours, sugar and salt in a mixing bowl. Rub in the margarine then add the dried yeast and mix well.
2. Mix in the water to make a soft dough.
3. Place the dough on a floured surface and knead well for at least 10 minutes, until firm and elastic and non-sticky.
4. Divide the dough in half, shape into rounds, then cover and leave in a warm place for at least 30 minutes or until doubled in size.
5. Place the dough rounds on a greased baking sheet and bake in a preheated oven at 230°C/450°F/gas mark 8 for 15 minutes. Reduce the heat to 200°C/400°F/gas mark 6 and cook for a further 20–30 minutes.
6. Cool on a wire rack.

SEED AND MUSTARD PLAIT

V | Ve

Makes 1

Metric/Imperial		American
350g/12oz	strong wholemeal flour	3 cups
350g/12oz	strong plain white flour	3 cups
2 tsp	celery salt	2 tsp
7g/¼oz	sachet easy-bake yeast	1 tbsp
4	spring onions, chopped	4
4 tbsp	pumpkin seeds	4 tbsp
4 tbsp	sunflower seeds	4 tbsp
1 tbsp	poppy seeds	1 tbsp
50ml/2 fl oz	olive oil	¼ cup
50ml/2fl oz	whole-grain mustard	3 tbsp
600ml/1 pint	hand-warm water	2½ cups
2½ tbsp	whole-grain mustard	2½ tbsp
1 tbsp	milk	1 tbsp
	extra seeds, for sprinkling	

1. Combine the flours, salt, yeast, onions and seeds in a bowl.
2. Mix the oil and water, stir in 2 tablespoons of the mustard and add to the dry mix, stirring well.
3. Turn onto a lightly floured surface and knead well for 5 minutes until smooth.
4. Divide into 3 pieces and shape into long ropes. Plait together and put on a greased baking sheet. Cover and leave in a warm place for 1 hour or until doubled in size.
5. Preheat oven to 200°C/400°F/gas mark 6.

Baking

6. Mix the milk with the remaining mustard and brush over the dough to glaze. Sprinkle with a few extra seeds.
7. Bake for 25–30 minutes until golden brown and firm.
8. Cool on a wire rack.

SEED BREAD

Makes 3

Metric/Imperial		American
25g/1oz	fresh yeast	2 tbsp
750ml/1¼ pints	hand-warm water	3¼ cups
1.4 kg/3 lb	wholewheat flour	3 lb
50g/2oz	poppy seeds	⅓ cup
50g/2oz	sesame seeds	⅓ cup
50g/2oz	sunflower seeds	⅓ cup
125ml/5fl oz	soya oil	⅔ cup
¼ tsp	salt	¼ tsp

1. Put yeast and water in a large bowl and mix until dissolved. Stir in enough flour to make a thick batter. Cover and leave in a warm place for 30 minutes.
2. Stir in the seeds, oil and salt, mix well and slowly add more flour, stirring constantly. When the dough begins to firm, place on a floured surface and knead. Add more flour until the consistency is smooth and elastic.
3. Return the dough to the bowl and leave in a warm place for 1 hour.
4. Gently knead the dough again, divide into 3 pieces and knead again briefly.
5. Fit the dough into 3 greased and floured 450g/1 lb bread tins, cover and leave to rise for 20–25 minutes.
6. Bake in the centre of a preheated oven at 230°C/450°F/gas mark 8 for 15 minutes. Reduce the heat to

180°C/350°F/gas mark 4 and bake for a further 30 minutes.

7. Remove from the tins and cool on a wire rack.

HIGH PROTEIN LOAF

Makes 1

Metric/Imperial		American
6	eggs, separated	6
1 tbsp	sesame seeds or caraway seeds	1 tbsp
½ tsp	salt	½ tsp
200g/8oz	soya flour, sifted	2 cups

1. Preheat oven to 180°C/350°F/gas mark 4.
2. Beat the egg yolks until very thick and pale. Add the seeds and salt.
3. Beat the egg whites until very stiff, then fold in the yolks. Add the flour to the mixture carefully folding in.
4. Pour the mixture into a buttered 1 kg/2.2 lb loaf tin.
5. Bake for 25 minutes, then reduce the heat to 130°C/250°F/gas mark ½ and bake for a further 15 minutes.
6. Remove from the tin and cool on a wire rack.

Note

This bread is rather crumbly with a fine sponge-like texture, but is delicious toasted.

The Glycaemic Index

This index can be seen as a scale for the conversion of foods to sugar in the blood. The blood sugar absorption and the subsequent level of sugar in our blood is influenced by many factors. These include the type of food that we eat, the fibre content of the food, the processing and cooking procedures and accompanying foods and drinks.

The glycaemic index provides useful clues to the manner in which various carbohydrate-rich foods influence our blood sugar. The diabetic food-exchange lists are based on the premise of calorie-equivalent portions. This system does not fully take into account the effects of food absorption on the blood sugar level. For instance, wheat will raise the blood sugar more than an equivalent amount of corn or rice.

The higher the index number the speedier the sugar effect on the blood, eg glucose is 100. Conversely the lower the number, the more appropriate the food for inclusion in a recipe for low blood sugar. This explains why complex carbohydrates are recommended but refined carbohydrate foods are not.

THE GLYCAEMIC INDEX

Sugars

Glucose	100
Honey	87
Sucrose	59
Fructose	20

Cereals

Cornflakes	80
Wholegrain bread	72
White rice	72
White bread	69
Brown rice	68
Shredded wheat	67
Swiss muesli	66
Sweetcorn	59
All bran	51
Spaghetti	50
Oatmeal cereal	49
Wholewheat spaghetti	42

Fruit

Raisins	64
Banana	62
Orange juice	46
Apple juice	45
Orange	40
Apple	39

Vegetables

Parsnip	97
Carrot	92
Mashed potato	80
Potato	70
Beetroot	64
Frozen peas	51
Peas	33

Pulses

Baked beans	40
Lima beans	36
Kidney beans	29
Lentils	29
Soya beans	15

Dairy Products

Yogurt (plain)	36
Ice cream	36
Whole milk	34
Skimmed milk	32

Various

Chocolate bar	68–75
Chips	51
Sponge cake	46
Peanuts	13

Product Information Services

Asda

Customer Services Dept, Asda House, Great Wilson
Street, Leeds LS11 5AD
Tel: 0113 1417730

Boots

Health and Nutrition Centre, The Boots Co plc,
Freepost, City Gate House, Nottingham MG2 3BR

Gateway

Customer Relations, Gateway House, Hawkfield
Business Park, Whitchurch Lane, Bristol BS14 0TJ

Marks and Spencer

Sue Chalk, Marks and Spencer, 47 Baker Street, London
W1A 1PN
Tel: 0171 268 6478

Safeway

Nutrition Advice Service, Safeway plc, 6 Millington Road, Hayes, Middx UB3 4AY

Sainsbury

Customer Services, J Sainsbury plc, Stamford House, Stamford Street, London SE1 9LL
Tel: 0171 921 6000

Tesco

The Nutritionist, Tesco, PO Box 18, Cheshunt, Herts EN8 9SL

Waitrose

Nutrition Advice Service, Waitrose, Southern Industrial Area, Bracknell, Berks RG12 4AY
Tel: 01344 424680

Further Reading

Airola, Paava. *Hypoglycaemia: A Better Approach*, Health Plus, 1977

Budd, Martin L. *Low Blood Sugar*, Thorsons, 1984

Budd, Martin L. *Diets to Help Diabetes*, Thorsons, 1994

Davis, Francyne. *The Low Blood Sugar Cookbook*, Bantam, 1974

Fredericks, Carlton. *New Low Blood Sugar and You*, Perigee, 1985

Hill, Diane. *Vegan Vitality*, Thorsons, 1987

Horsley, Janet. *Sugar-free Cookbook*, Prism Press, 1993

Scott, David. *Protein-rich Vegetarian Cookery*, Rider, 1985

Scuthering & Lousley. *Diabetic Delights*, Martin Dunitz, 1986

Wakeman & Baskerville. *The Vegan Cookbook*, Faber & Faber, 1986

COOKING TERMS

British	*American*
Aubergine	Eggplant
Baking tray	Cookie sheet
Bicarbonate of soda	Baking soda
Biscuits, savoury	Crackers
Biscuits, sweet	Cookies
Black olives	Ripe olives
Broad beans	Fava beans, or use lima beans
Butter muslin	Cheesecloth
Cake mixture	Cake batter
Cake tin	Cake pan
Chicory	Belgian endive
Cocktail stick	Toothpick
Cornflour	Cornstarch
Cos lettuce	Romaine
Courgettes	Zucchini
Curly endive	Chicory
Digestive biscuits	Use graham crackers
Double cream	Heavy/whipping cream
Essence	Extract
Frying pan	Skillet
Grated rind	Grated zest or peel
Greaseproof paper	Waxed paper
Grill/grilled	Broil/broiled
Groundnut oil	Peanut oil
Gruyère cheese	Swiss cheese
Haricot beans	Navy beans
Heart of lettuce	Bulk of Boston lettuce

Low Blood Sugar

Maize flour	Corn meal
Mange tout	Snow peas
Marrow	Large zucchini/marrow squash
Mixture	Batter
Porridge oats	Rolled/quick cooking oats
Scones	Biscuits
Single cream	Light cream
Soya beans	Soybeans
Spring onion	Scallion
Stoned	Pitted
Sultanas	Golden raisins
Wholewheat plain flour	Whole-wheat flour
Wholewheat self-raising flour	Whole-wheat flour sifted with baking powder
Yeast, dried	Active-dry yeast
Yeast, fresh	Compressed yeast

General Index

Recipe Index

Low Blood Sugar